THE CLINICIAN'S GUIDE TO GERIATRIC FORENSIC EVALUATIONS

THE CLINICIAN'S GUIDE TO GERIATRIC FORENSIC EVALUATIONS

KAREN REIMERS
Adjunct Assistant Professor
Department of Psychiatry
University of Minnesota
Minneapolis, MN
United States

ELSEVIER

ACADEMIC PRESS
An imprint of Elsevier

Academic Press is an imprint of Elsevier
125 London Wall, London EC2Y 5AS, United Kingdom
525 B Street, Suite 1650, San Diego, CA 92101, United States
50 Hampshire Street, 5th Floor, Cambridge, MA 02139, United States
The Boulevard, Langford Lane, Kidlington, Oxford OX5 1GB, United Kingdom

Library of Congress Cataloging-in-Publication Data
A catalog record for this book is available from the Library of Congress

British Library Cataloguing-in-Publication Data
A catalogue record for this book is available from the British Library

ISBN: 978-0-12-815034-4

For information on all Academic Press publications visit our website at https://www.elsevier.com/books-and-journals

Publisher: Nikki Levy
Acquisition Editor: Nikki Levy
Editorial Project Manager: Michelle W. Fisher
Production Project Manager: Bharatwaj Varatharajan
Cover Designer: Miles Hitchen

Typeset by TNQ Technologies

To my grandparents, whose sacrifices and hard work allowed me to follow my ambitions.

Contents

Preface

An 84-year-old woman hospitalized for treatment of pneumonia. After a few days of antibiotics, the treatment team feels she ready for discharge alone to her home, from a medical standpoint. However, her daughter has discovered unpaid bills and two full bottles of her mother's medications. The patient's Folstein Mini-Mental State Examination (MMSE) score is 26/30. Her daughter and discharge planner wonder if it is safe for patient to return home. Her doctor is uncertain how to determine the patient's decision-making capacity.

As clinicians, we are often tasked with evaluating older individuals about questions at the interface of law, medicine, and psychiatry. Whether we realize it or not, geriatric forensic evaluations are part of everyday practice for all of us working with older adults — regardless of if we are physicians including psychiatrists, psychologists, or other advanced practice clinicians. Many important forensic issues are faced every day by older patients across almost all medical specialties and settings. Capacity to consent to treatment is one of the most common questions faced in the clinical context, but capacity to drive, manage finances or live independently are also very common.

Courts frequently call upon psychiatric and other forensic clinicians to help them understand and interpret information about decision-making capacity and a range of other medico-legal topics. There are many reasons why elders might be involved with the courts, including issues related to decision-making capacity, criminal questions, inheritance and will contests, contracts, torts, real estate, guardianship, Social Security, protected tenancy, family, labor, evidence, tax, bankruptcy, and banking (Doron et al., 2017). Geriatric forensic evaluations can carry far reaching consequences for older adults, and stakes are often high — for a finding of incapacity can strip an individual of his or her individual rights, leading the older adult to lose more rights than a convicted felon. Court findings of incapacity or need for guardianship can be very difficult to overturn.

By 2050, the 65-and-older demographic will rise to about ¼ of the U.S. population. Across modern industrialized democracies, populations are fortunate to enjoy good health, leading to a longer lifespan. Aging of the population is bringing new societal phenomena, including elderly individuals caring for their own parents, marriages at older ages, and professionals working much longer than in previous generations. This brings both challenges and exciting new possibilities for society.

The sizeable Baby Boomer generation is now moving into late adulthood—and this cohort does not intend to go quietly. New phenomena with the Boomer generation include longer lifespan, but also higher rates of substance abuse, increasing divorce rates, increasing single-person households, and issues related to mixed/blended families, such as complex estate plan structures with multiple stepchildren. The posthumous redistribution of wealth for the Boomer generation will be of unparalleled magnitude. At the same time, many Baby Boomers have not saved enough for retirement, and are often finding that unusual demands are placed upon them, as the incomes of the next generation are not up to par. Compared with previous generations, Boomers are increasingly asked to make loans to family, while having a desire to not be dependent on their children in the future, and hoping to have enough money to last to the end of their life.

Increasing rates of dementia and other neurocognitive disorders in the aging population complicate the evaluation and treatment of a growing number of individuals. Dementia and neurocognitive disorders affect core areas of civil and criminal forensic practice - especially capacity questions, including competence to stand trial and criminal responsibility, vulnerability to undue influence, and many others.

Unfortunately, many clinicians have little or no training in proper forensic assessment and evaluation techniques, or on factors germane to the geriatric population such as evaluation of cognitive impairment. Ageism, lack of knowledge, and practical challenges can lead to incompetence on the part of a geriatric forensic evaluator. It is complicated to apply a universal template in every forensic situation, since rules vary by jurisdiction - so local convention, gut feeling, and efficiency considerations may prevail over competent evaluation techniques. Clinician evaluators may rely excessively on screening tests such as Mini-Mental State Examination (MMSE) scores, leading to shoddy diagnosis of Alzheimer's with potentially terrible consequences for the older individual. In some of the hospitals and clinics where we practice, institutional policies or interdisciplinary collaboration may shield the clinical treatment provider from some of the forensic and decision-making work - for example, social workers and occupational therapists are involved with determinations of capacity to live independently after discharge from inpatient care. Collaboration with forensic colleagues or independent forensic evaluators can certainly be helpful, but resource limitations in most settings and the fast pace of modern medicine often means such services are underutilized.

As a result, many clinicians are hesitant to get involved with legal questions, and this area can be quite stressful and difficult for clinicians to navigate. In general, those of us who diagnose and treat older adults tend to be skeptical and anxious about interacting with the legal system, preoccupied with the threat of medical malpractice litigation, and disparaging of "ambulance chasers."

Nevertheless, as clinicians we can benefit from improving our knowledge and skills in geriatric forensic evaluations. Many skills are necessary for successful geriatric forensic practice, including the abilities to conduct a productive examination of the older person, distil the most important and relevant information from a large quantity of data, and process the information obtained in a rational manner, to answer the legal questions posed.

Adding to the complexity of geriatric forensic evaluations, the Diagnostic and Statistical Manual of Mental Disorders fifth Edition (DSM-5) (APA, 2013) introduced new concepts of diagnosis which may seem bewildering to clinicians tasked with evaluating geriatric individuals, especially for those who trained under the older diagnostic system. Executive function is a key neuropsychological concept to understand and, at times, formal neuropsychological assessment can be a critical part of determining the extent of actual cognitive changes including the subtler presentations such as mild cognitive disorder that can affect key questions of need for guardianship or capacity for decision-making in different domains.

Despite the increasing numbers of older people in our society, the number of publications in geriatric forensic psychiatry is lacking. Until recently, special considerations for older adults, particularly dementia and cognitive impairment, were rarely addressed in the literature about adult forensic evaluations. One enduring exception has been the outstanding Psychologist's Guide to Assessment of Older Adults with Diminished Capacity (ABA and APA, 2008), which remains a seminal resource for clinicians working in this area. Beyond this however, around the time I began researching this subject in 2016, the last major publication by a psychiatrist on the topic of geriatric forensic psychiatry had been published in 1987, about 30 years prior. (Rosner and Schwartz, 1987)

Through my own clinical experiences, particularly working as an adult psychiatrist in rural Wisconsin conducting court-ordered independent psychiatric evaluations for civil commitment, re-commitment, and guardianship, I became increasingly interested in the interface of civil legal questions and clinical psychiatry. To improve my clinical and forensic practice with older adults, I started to check the available resources to guide clinicians in conducting geriatric forensic evaluations, and was surprised at how few reference materials were available specifically about older adults and the legal system. The idea for this book came from this relative dearth of practical resources about forensic evaluations in older adults. The book's outline is based on lecture I presented on Geriatric Forensic Evaluations at the 2017 Midwest Chapter Annual Meeting of the American Academy for Psychiatry and the Law in Kansas City, MO. Since then, exciting developments in the field of geriatric forensic evaluations include the publication of the groundbreaking comprehensive textbook Geriatric Forensic Psychiatry: Principles and Practice (Holzer et al., 2018) and expansion of the psychology literature in this area, including another recent textbook Forensic Geropsychology: Practice Essentials (Bush and Heck, 2017).

In this book, clinicians will discover that many geriatric forensic evaluation approaches and techniques can be learned and applied. This book is intended for psychiatrists including general adult psychiatrists, forensic psychiatrists, and geriatric psychiatrists. It may also be of interest to psychologists and family medicine providers who make capacity determinations as part of their clinical practice.

As our population ages, the importance of geriatric forensic evaluations is growing. Given the dearth of specialists in geriatric forensic psychiatry at a time when we are facing rapid increase in the need for specialized expertize in this area, I hope this book will offer a useful introductory guide to clinicians conducting geriatric forensic evaluations.

Objectives of this book

1. Explore how geriatric forensic evaluations differ from general adult forensic evaluations including practical, ethical, and legal considerations
2. List forensic assessment techniques for older adults, and common pitfalls
3. Identify helpful practices for gathering geriatric forensic information and use of collateral information

Chapter-by-chapter summary

With a focus on providing guidance to the practicing clinician, each chapter of this book highlights key points for clinicians and key references for further learning.

Chapter 1 provides a general introduction to the geriatric forensic evaluation and highlights how geriatric forensic evaluations differ from general forensic evaluations. Many factors make evaluation of an elderly individual different from a young person including the role of complex medical factors, medications, generational questions and ethical considerations. The chapter reviews key components of the mental status exam.

Chapter 2 reviews ethical and legal considerations including criminal aspects of geriatric forensic evaluations.

Chapter 3 covers evaluation of cognition in older adults, the cognitive changes in normal aging, criteria for diagnosing dementia, mild cognitive impairment, and DSM-5 neurocognitive disorders for the practicing clinician.

Chapter 4 provides an overview of capacity evaluations. Clinicians in a variety of settings including primary care and outpatient psychiatric practice are asked to assess elderly patients for capacity on a daily basis, for capacity to consent to treatment, driving capacity, capacity to live independently, and less frequently for testamentary capacity (ability to make a valid will) and other questions. The chapter also discusses surrogate decision-making and evaluations for guardianship.

Chapter 5 discusses elder abuse, elder financial exploitation, and undue influence. Elder abuse is a huge and growing problem, vastly underreported and it is something that clinicians treating older people in every setting will encounter. Undue influence is a legal concept but psychiatrists have unique expertize in evaluating an older person's vulnerability to coercion or manipulation.

Chapter 6 reviews best practices, problems and pitfalls for geriatric forensic report writing and testimony. These expert communications can help the judge and/or jury arrive at a legal conclusion.

The Afterword offers a view into the future of geriatric forensic evaluations, highlighting key emerging topics likely to have a major impact on the field and on the future of millions of older adults.

Appendices include an interview template, sample reports, and the Montreal Cognitive Assessment (MoCA) examination.

Conclusion

All of us are aging, and it is in our collective interest to promote competence in geriatric forensic evaluations. These questions could apply to any of us in the future. Though it is sometimes challenging, it is also rewarding and meaningful for clinicians to develop the skills to assist elders in this way. I hope this book can serve as a starting guide and resource for all clinicians involved with evaluating older individuals for forensic purposes.

REFERENCES

American Bar Association and American Psychological Association, 2008. Assessment of Older Adults with Diminished Capacity: A Handbook for Psychologists. ABA/APA, Washington, DC.

American Psychiatric Association, 2013. Diagnostic and statistical manual of mental disorders fifth ed. Arlington, VA.

Bush, S., Heck, A. (Eds.), 2018. Forensic Geropsychology: Practice Essentials.

Doron, I.I., Werner, P., Spanier, B., Lazar, O., 2017. The legal appearances of dementia in court rulings: mapping the terrain. Int. Psychogeriatr. 1–9.

Holzer, J.C., Kohn, R., Ellison, J.M., Recupero, P.R., 2018. Geriatric Forensic Psychiatry: Principles and Practice. Oxford University Press, New York, NY.

Rosner, R., Schwartz, H.I., 1987. Geriatric Psychiatry and the Law. Plenum Press.

Acknowledgments

Writing a book is a team effort. I am especially thankful to the editors and staff at Elsevier, particularly Michelle Fisher, Carlos Rodriguez, Bharatwaj Varatharajan, Sheela Josy and Nikki Levy for providing me with the opportunity to publish this book and for their professional guidance. Thanks also to my personal administrative and research assistants Laurie Kaplan, Victoria Acuna, Susan Fritz, Morgan Province, Kristina Radovic, Harwinder Singh, Jason Slizgi, Donna Stannard, and Slimani Zied.

Thank you to my valued professional colleagues who provided mentorship and encouragement to learn about clinical, geriatric and forensic issues over the years: Belito Arana, David Atkinson, Steve Babitsky, Natasha Cervantes, David Conn, George Dawson, Bradleigh Dornfeld, Sanford Finkel, Chinmoy Gulrajani, Wilson Igbrude, Ian Lamoureux, Bob Lawson, Nick Mathew, Paul Newhouse, Bill Orr, sponsors of the 2012 AAGP Partners HealthCare Honors Scholarship, Mark Rapoport, Jim Reynolds, Phil Resnick, Tatyana Shteinlukht, Sherif Soliman, and Ilse Wiechers.

Finally, a big thank you to my family and friends for all their care and support.

Disclaimer

All patient names mentioned in the book are fictitious and any similarity to real individuals is purely coincidental and unintentional.

CHAPTER ONE

Introduction to geriatric forensic evaluations

Contents

The Clinician's Guide to Geriatric Forensic Evaluations
ISBN: 978-0-12-815034-4
https://doi.org/10.1016/B978-0-12-815034-4.00001-5

An elderly motorist turned into a bicyclist and killed him. The motorist kept on going to the grocery store, and never looked back. Driving back home a few minutes later, he encountered the scene of his own accident. Traffic was stopped while the police processed the scene. The motorist got out of his car, approached police, and started cursing and yelling that they were keeping him from getting home with his groceries. A bystander pointed him out as the same motorist who killed the victim a few minutes before. The motorist was arrested, and he was later deemed incompetent to proceed. His driver's license was revoked.

(Reynolds, 2016).

Our aging population will bring new opportunities and challenges for both medicine and the law. Geriatric forensic evaluations evaluate older people in a legal context Forensic psychiatric experts play an important role in assisting legal decision-makers.

This chapter will provide an introduction to geriatric forensic evaluations. A psychiatric clinician who is experienced in working with older adults is in a position to assist attorneys, courts, regulators, other clinicians, caregivers, and families with issues at the interface of the law and psychiatry.

Who are older adults?

How should we define "geriatric"? Age 65 is often used as a cutoff, however if "geriatric" is defined by frailty, cognitive impairment, or dependence, then most 65-year-olds today do not qualify. Many individuals are very healthy, active, independent, mentally sharp, and vibrant well into their 80s and 90s. They do not fit the conventional idea of "geriatric". In contrast, we see early "geriatric" features in certain subpopulations including incarcerated individuals. Some studies classify older adults starting at age 49 due to the accelerated aging seen in those settings due to a combination of factors including lifestyle, stress, poor diet, substance abuse, and others. The "very old" - individuals 85 and older - are growing at the fastest rate. This will bring some social, health, and economic consequences. (Shulman, 2018).

Clinical judgment rules the day about whether a person is considered to be "older" for the purposes of evaluation techniques, and this may depend on the clinician's assessment of the person's cognitive, social, and medical vulnerabilities. Aging is a continuum, so there is not necessarily a clearly defined demarcation. Overall, it is difficult to envision one "characteristic" older person as a representative of the entire group. Factors, such as age (especially over age 85), mental health, physical health, and social supports differentiate one older individual from another.

Older individuals are very diverse; they are not a homogeneous group.

Ageism and older adults

Many individuals in society still view older people as infirm, feeble, and incapable while older people often see themselves as younger, fit, and capable. Evaluators should be conscious of their own potentially ageist biases. They should be careful not to sound patronizing or to classify older people in their mind as incapable. They should recognize that many conditions are treatable in old age and not assume that "nothing can be done (Erber and Szuchman, 2014)."

Beware of ageism and false generational assumptions.

What are forensic evaluations?

The term "forensic" is often used to describe the use of science to investigate crime. However, the term "forensic" used in "forensic psychiatry" refers to the application of psychiatry to the law, and to psychiatric treatment in forensic (legal) settings, such as courts, jails, and prisons.

There are more civil than criminal questions where geriatric forensic evaluations are required, including guardianship assessment of testamentary and other capacities. Forensic questions pertaining to older people include issues like legal cognitive capacity, competence to be tried or enter a plea, be a witness, give general consent, and enter a contract. Forensic evaluators are tasked with determining if a brain disorder interferes with an individual's capacity to understand, decide on, or act in a specific circumstance before the law (Holzer et al., 2018).

What is forensic psychiatry?

As defined by the American Academy of Psychiatry and the Law (AAPL):

Forensic psychiatry is a medical subspecialty that includes research and clinical practice in the many areas in which psychiatry is applied to legal issues. While some forensic psychiatrists may specialize exclusively in legal issues, almost all psychiatrists may, at some point, have to work within one of the many areas in which the mental health and legal system overlap.

AAPL, 2018

Forensic interviewing

The definition of forensic interviewing has taken decades to develop. There are many different types of questions that can be explored with a forensic interview including criminal questions, civil questions of capacity and guardianship evaluations, civil commitment proceedings, and interviewing victims of crime including elder abuse.

Defining Forensic Interviewing

A forensic interview ... is a developmentally sensitive and legally sound method of gathering factual information [...] This interview is conducted by a competently trained, neutral professional utilizing research and practice-informed techniques as part of a larger investigative process.

OJJDP, 2015

Who performs geriatric forensic evaluations?

Forensic interviews are best conducted within the context of a multidisciplinary team. They may include many different individuals, each with something unique to contribute. By the time you, as a mental health professional, are seated in an interview room with an older adult, many other people and/or professions have already become directly involved with that individual and their case. Usefulness of the process, in terms of multidisciplinary teams, is directly dependent on allowing the abilities of that older adult to be maximized in order to elicit factual information regarding that individual's experience. Many people have an interest in the process and particularly of what the outcome will be.

Clinicians acting in an expert role in geriatric forensic evaluations have a unique part to play. They must step outside of the usual parameters of the confidential physician-patient relationship in a variety of ways. They may share information with courts and lawyers. They must maintain a neutral attitude toward the interview. If the examinee needs treatment, they will refer colleagues to avoid potential conflicts of interest. The goal is to answer the psychiatric question as objectively as possible.

Possible self-identities of forensic report writers:

- Scientist Clinician
- Investigator
- Journalist-reporter
- Quasi-attorney
- Judicial decision-maker
- Court educator
- Businessperson
- Health care administrator
- Artist -writer
- Policy advocate

Buchanan and Norko, 2011

It is important to note that for civil questions (such as capacity assessment), clinicians may find themselves involved in a dual role, testifying to the court as an expert about a patient under their clinical care. Ideally, an independent forensic evaluator would address legal questions while the clinician would focus on the medical treatment. Mixing clinical and forensic roles can at times lead to conflicts and ethical dilemmas, and ergo compromising both roles. However, a total separation of clinical and forensic realms is not possible, particularly in the civil arena.

Geriatric-specific legal rules and procedures can vary considerably by jurisdiction, even among US jurisdictions. For any specific case where a geriatric forensic evaluation is required, experts must communicate with retaining counsel to clearly define the key legal questions and criteria to be addressed in the geriatric forensic evaluation and report.

Multidisciplinary team

In clinical settings, geriatric care is often a team effort. Eventually, a team approach could also be applied more formally to geriatric forensic evaluations. At this time, collaboration in clinical settings often appears limited to relying on support staff for collateral information, particularly in retrospective evaluations when reviewing nursing home records when evaluating testamentary capacity. Collaboration with neuropsychologists is an important area.

Members of a multidisciplinary team for geriatric forensic interviews can include:

- Law enforcement and emergency medical personnel
- Adult protective services
- Mental health professionals
- Medical providers
- Nursing facility staff
- Financial professionals
- Family, neighbors and friends
- Prosecuting and defending attorneys

The role of informants and collateral is very different for forensic versus the clinical evaluation where we would normally rely on collateral intake information at face value. For forensic questions, informants and collateral sources may have secondary involvement or gain, which would make them bias. This could be involvement in capacity evaluation, testamentary capacity, financial abuse or public interest situations (Holzer et al., 2018).

Existing guidelines for geriatric forensic evaluations

With regards to the mechanics of the evaluation itself, there are many considerations specific to older individuals. At this time, there is very limited information in existing guidelines about specific techniques for geriatric evaluations in the general psychiatric evaluation.

The American Psychological Association did, however, publish specific guidelines on the psychological evaluation of older adults. (APA, 2014). Other sources focus primarily on younger adults but do offer somewhat more guidance on forensic evaluation of older people. (Heilbrun et al., 2009) (Gold and Vanderpool, 2013) (Pachana et al., 2011).

Guidelines for forensic evaluations

- The American Psychological Association's *Guidelines for Forensic Evaluation* (Association, 2013)
- The American Academy for Psychiatry and the Law's *Guidelines for Insanity Defense* (Janofsky, MD et al., 2014).
- The American Psychiatric Association's *General Adult Evaluation Guidelines* (APA Work Group on Psychiatric Evaluation, Silverman et al., 2016).
- The American Academy for Psychiatry and the Law's *Forensic Evaluation Guidelines* (Glancy et al., 2015).
- The American Academy for Psychiatry and the Law's *Competence to Stand Trial* Guidelines (Mossman et al., 2007)
- American Psychiatric Association's *Guidelines for Disability Evaluations* (Gold et al., 2008).

Types of geriatric forensic evaluations

There are many types of forensic evaluations. They can be classified into criminal or civil, contemporaneous or retrospective geriatric forensic evaluations.

Criminal geriatric forensic evaluations

Competence to stand trial and insanity defense are the mainstays of criminal forensic evaluations that are often ordered by the courts. These two types of evaluations and other issues for geriatric offenders are discussed in more detail in Chapter 2.

Adjudicative process

Within the criminal justice system, there are many features pertinent to the increasing aging population including elder abuse, neglect, financial exploitation, and the increase in elderly criminal defendants. Elderly persons appear in criminal court most frequently as victims of crime, not perpetrators. However, there has also been an increase in elderly offenders. Many challenges are presented working with an elderly defendant through the adjudicative process.

Elements of the adjudicative process.

- Point of arrest
- booking
- initial hearing
- arraignment
- discovery and trial
- plea negotiations
- disposition
- appeal

Wall, 2018; Holzer et al., 2018

Malingering/feigning

Occasionally, forensic clinicians encounter referrals for competence evaluations that seem frivolous, because the defendant is obviously competent. Clinicians should recognize, however, that when a defendant displays signs of a competence-impairing mental disorder, defense counsel is obligated to question whether the client can proceed with adjudication. (Glancy et al., 2015).

Because of the severe consequences of a malingering finding of the defendant, psychiatrists should not make this diagnosis lightly. Solid evidence, not clinical suspicion, should be the basis of such a determination (Glancy et al., 2015). On the other hand, the benefit of a defendant successfully convincing the evaluator and court that he or she is incompetent could mean a delayed trial, accommodations other than jail until the trial, and/or a more lenient sentence. For many, these outcomes are worth feigning incompetence. If the psychiatrist suspects malingering but do not have sufficient evidence to make that diagnosis, he or she can recommend that the defendant enter an inpatient unit where around-the-clock observation can help confirm or deny the charge of malingering (Glancy et al., 2015).

Potential sources of confirmatory evidence of malingering:

- Psychological testing or specialized instruments for detecting malingering
- Medical, psychological, and/or custodial records
- Interviews with family, friends, police, custodial officers, and others who have had contact with the defendant
- History with the criminal justice system

Glancy et al., 2015

Civil geriatric forensic evaluations

For most clinicians, civil questions are the bulk of geriatric forensic evaluations. There are many issues to consider. They include capacity assessment in various settings, civil commitments for inpatient, outpatient, and nursing home, and many others. These questions are discussed in subsequent chapters.

Contemporaneous geriatric forensic evaluations

This is the most common type of evaluation in geriatric forensic psychiatry. It involves assessment of the older person during her or his lifetime, usually by clinical interview.

Retrospective geriatric forensic evaluations

This type of evaluation, more common with questions of testamentary capacity or undue influence, occurs after the individual is deceased. The forensic evaluator will conduct a historical reconstruction, piece together the available facts to see whether the shed light on the person's mental functioning at a specific point in the past.

How do geriatric forensic evaluations differ from forensic evaluations in younger people?

General Considerations

Many elements are similar to techniques used with younger adults, however, older people have increased the potential for cognitive problems. Older adults may have issues with sensory input, hearing, and vision issues that can have a negative impact on their ability to provide or understand important information. Difficulties may be obvious as the evaluation gets started. Cognitive and sensory problems can make an older person appear confused. There may also be chronic and/or acute psychiatric, medical, and/or neurological health problems. These can affect attention, memory, language, mood, perception, and/or behavior. Medications are an especially important source of potential problems for mental functioning.

Techniques for Evaluating Older Adults

- Ask open-ended questions first, then use process-of-elimination questions
- Later, ask more specific questions rather than broad questions
- Listen patiently and redirect as needed if the older adult digresses
- Use memory cues such as "What were you doing before this happened?"
- Do not discount the entire interview because the older adult has made statements that seem untrue or may be the result of delusions

Gibson, 2017

Clinicians will also want to limit using infantilizing language with older adults, not calling the person "Honey" or "Sweetie" or talking to them in a tone as would be used with children. Many professionals do this unconsciously, but it has an important impact on the older adult who is being evaluated, and it should be avoided (Gibson, 2017).

Performing a comprehensive interview with an older adult in distress can be a daunting task. The additional stress of a forensic evaluation adds even more difficulty. Multiple interviews may be needed, especially when it comes to questions of mild cognitive impairment, which can take time to assess (Wang et al., 2017). Older adults have a lifetime of experiences as well as ailments and impediments of old age. Often, they have limited ability to summarize their history accurately and collecting the most important information requires a skilled interviewer. To develop this skill, remember that it is impossible to generate a complete differential diagnosis and comprehensive summary in a short time.

Evaluators should take the time to familiarize themselves with older people person's background and be sure to understand the relationship of the older person with their family.

Obtain as much background information as possible before the interview and review available records. It is important to have a clear understanding of why the patient is visiting today, with whom, and the specific legal question and criteria that need to be addressed. It may be helpful to ask the older adults or their collateral informant to complete questionnaires or intake packets prior to the interview. If possible, collect collateral information from the patient's caregivers or other relevant collateral sources. Depending on the legal question, collateral information may focus on prior school, military, and occupational history and records.

A thoughtful review of diagnostic testing should also occur as part of the evaluation. You should consider: [1] underlying disease processes and cognitive deficits, [2] laboratory tests, [3] imaging studies, and [3] neurological, neuropsychological and/or psychological testing (Holzer et al., 2018).

The legal questions related to the case can guide the history, exam, and collateral information that need to be obtained. Factors, which are salient to the legal question and/or legal standard, should be highlighted by the examiner. Prior forensic or legal history including [1] prior mental health conditions, [2] civil commitment, [3] criminal competence, and [4] guardianship should be obtained via a records review in advance (Holzer et al., 2018).

Historical elements may relate directly to the current legal issue. A detailed personal history can include a history of abuse and trauma, as well as, developmental, educational, occupational, military, and social aspects. Family history should include not only medical and psychiatric family history but also clinical and legal issues, which may support and/or conflict within the family. Overall, the different types of histories should be tailored to the legal context.

A well-planned forensic assessment of a geriatric person requires neural medical psychiatric examination techniques. These include exam, lab testing, structural neuroimaging, cognitive screening, and neuropsychological testing. It may also involve lumbar puncture, functional neuroimaging, or other medical examinations (Holzer et al., 2018).

Mechanics of the evaluation

An elderly person may have difficulties with transportation, walking, or getting to a particular evaluation locale. Determine the best time of day to conduct the interview. Mornings are generally best since many older adults tend to be more aware and alert earlier in the day. Some older adults with dementia may experience sun-downing, so evenings or afternoons are not optimal.

You must also consider accessibility needs that include assistive devices, such as walkers, wheelchairs, and/or canes. Collaboration with health care providers regarding transport, emergency shelter placement, medication management and making sure that they have hearing aids, dentures, and/or eyeglasses might also be an important part of that process.

Mobility Issues
- Conduct interview in the best location for the older adult
- Consider future needs for transportation and accessibility at police station and court
- Arrange for assistive devices if needed
- Collaborate with health care providers

The site and timing of evaluation can affect the evaluation process. Difficulties in transportation can be a problem, and public transportation may be more accessible than other ways of transport for meetings and clinical office work. Ambulation may be a difficulty. Evaluations that are conducted in the late afternoon or evening might more likely to uncover cognitive deficits due to fatigue or sun-downing.

Addressing sensory input deficits

Older individuals suffer from an increased prevalence of medical problems, which include: [1] fatigue, [2] decreased concentration, [3] poor hearing, and [4] diminished eyesight. Although many of these conditions are treatable, they should not be underestimated.

Evaluators should ensure that hearing aids and glasses are available and used.

Impairments and accommodations
- Vision – glasses, large text, magnifier
- Gait – walker, wheelchair
- Hearing – hearing aids, pocket talker

Communication techniques

Possible barriers to disclosure
- Communication skills
- Comprehension skills
- Developmental disability
- Impaired cognitive functioning
- Number of prior abuse discussions can make an elderly person just not want to talk about it anymore.
- Language shame

Possible barriers to disclosure ***(cont'd)***

- Embarrassment, guilt, culpability or self-blame
- Emotional or physical threats from the perpetrator
- Fear of losing one's independence
- Secrecy
- Loyalty and/or protection of the perpetrator
- Family privacy protection
- Cultural issues such as: gender, race, ethnicity, socioeconomic status and/or religion
- Competency such as: emotional status, developmental disabilities and/or cognitive functioning

Gibson, 2017

Helpful interview strategies with older adults

- Establish the older adult's daily routine
- Construct each subsequent question building on what the older person has already told you
- Use the older adult's exact words or phrases.

Gibson, 2017

Ways enhance communication:

- Ask the older adult how he or she would prefer to communicate with you
- Ask how he or she prefers to be addressed (first or last name, Dr., Reverend?)
- Read written materials to the individual
- Use an interpreter if needed
- Use visual aids, charts, or diagrams
- Ask short questions
- Limit environmental distractions

Gibson, 2017

You may need to spend more time explaining the evaluation process to an older person and gaining their trust before the evaluation can proceed.

Communication strategies

- TALK tactics: Take it slow, Ask simple questions, Limit reality checks and Keep eye contact
- Approach from the front
- Introduce yourself
- Speak slowly
- Use simple, familiar language
- Ask one question/give one direction at a time
- Be mindful of body language
- Minimize distractions

Gibson, 2017

The importance of clear communication and adapting your communication style to older adults cannot be overstated. Here are some key points to follow:

- Always make sure that the person has their eyeglasses and/or hearing aids. You may want to keep a couple of reader glasses on hand or carry a pocket talker, which can help with communication. The only downside to a pocket talker is that it can't mute external noise. When it enhances noise, it enhances all the noise, so it's even more important to make sure that there are no distractions in the immediate environment.
- Select an appointment time that works well for the patient's daily routine. Patients with cognitive impairment frequently have worse performance later in the day. Late afternoon or evening appointments should be avoided. Mid-morning is often best.
- Make sure that the interview setting is quiet, private, and free of distractions that may disorient or upset the patient and impair his or her ability to participate.
- Perform a sensory check. Always be aware of sensory impairment, especially hearing and visual loss. If a patient does not answer your questions, consider whether he or she just might not be able to hear you. When hearing impairment is a factor, always speak loudly into the better ear. You may want to have an amplifying headset available for the patient (see Text Box). Ensure patients have their glasses so they can see adequately. Physical contact may be useful for the visually impaired.
- Establishing rapport is important. It is important to avoid confrontation and take measures to facilitate the evaluation and maximize that quality of information obtained (Holzer et al., 2018).

- To build rapport with patient and collateral source, consider if it is appropriate to smile.
- Maintain good eye contact.
- Use a soothing, yet audible, the tone of voice.
- Inquire about the patient's life history and family.
- Listen to the patient in a relaxed manner.
- Solicit questions and answer all of them.
- Do not rush questions. Be patient and wait for delayed responses.
- For patients with cognitive impairment, use simply worded questions with a single idea (i.e. Do you feel sad? Are you afraid?). Questions might need to be yes/no rather than open-ended.
- Provide language translation when necessary.

Several excellent books offer more detail about effective communication with older people, including older adults with dementia. (Agronin, 2014) (Coste, 2003) (Mace and Rabins, 2017) (Solie, 2004).

Using a "Pocket Talker" or other amplification device

Hearing enhancement devices such as a "Pocket Talker" are small portable personal sound amplifiers with a microphone. Such devices can help the forensic examiner achieve clear and loud delivery of speech without having to yell at the older person.

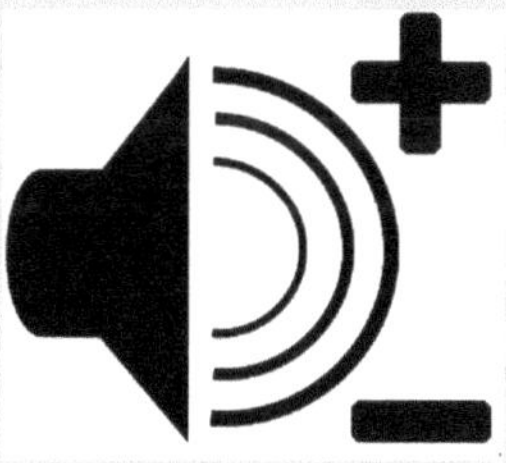

From https://svgsilh.com/image/1319376.html

Should you video record the evaluation?

The pros and cons of video or audio taping interviews with the defendant or plaintiff have been discussed in an AAPL task force report (AAPL, 1999), and elsewhere (Buchanan and Norko, 2011). Some of the advantages include being able to review the details of the interviews as part of preparation immediately prior to trial. With major crimes, trials may occur several years after the event or evaluation. Recordings also allow for a more accurate quotation of statements made by the defendant.

One of the cons is at the opposing side may also use them to prepare cross-examination questions. Another is that personal information not directly relevant to the case may be more available. Such tapes, in addition, to verifying what was said to the expert can become part of the public record and play in the national press.

The use of such aids to note-taking and record keeping should be reviewed with the retaining attorney and the defendant notified in advance, when feasible. Occasionally, in testamentary capacity evaluations, those hoping to demonstrate the capacity of a testator will record video, in an effort to show that they were cognitively intact or that their will was a reflection of their independent and capable wishes. Unfortunately, the naïve interviewer can often make the mistake of confusing the preservation of social graces for intact cognition and might consider passive acquiescence as evidence of independence of mind. Clinicians understand or should understand, that significant cognitive impairment can be readily missed if specific cognitions are not probed directly. A video of a testator is only as good as the skill of the interviewer and quality of the interview. In some cases, the video may inadvertently demonstrate the exact opposite of what was intended (Shulman, 2018).

Potentially reversible issues: medical, affective, social-context

An incorrect diagnosis of Alzheimer's disease can have far-reaching negative consequences for an older person. It is critically important to consider reversible causes of dementia and to rule these out. Dementia is frequently a diagnosis of exclusion. As many as 1 in 10 patients with dementia have a potentially reversible cause that should not be overlooked. Often, delirium may be superimposed on dementia. Moreover, the delirium can take weeks to resolve.

Evaluating the medical causes of cognitive problems needs careful assessment, often over a period of time. Medical causes of dementia-like syndromes can include: [1] hypothyroidism, [2] a vitamin B12 deficiency, [3] normal pressure hydrocephalus, [4] a brain tumor, [5] depression, [6] alcoholism, [7] an infection, [8] a subdural hematoma, [9] trauma, [10] anoxia, and/or [11] medication (Rosner, 2017). Intoxication and withdrawal syndromes are increasingly common, especially with the aging baby boomer generation.

Routine laboratory testing as part of the evaluation of suspected major neurocognitive disorders

- Complete blood count (CBC)
- Comprehensive metabolic panel (CMP)
- Thyroid stimulating hormone (TSH)
- Vitamin B12 and folate levels
- Rapid plasma reagin (RPR)

Mood problems, particularly depression, can mimic dementia causing a "pseudodementia" syndrome that resolves when depression is adequately treated. Therefore, careful assessment of the examinee's psychiatric status is critical. Moreover, social and contextual factors can cause an older individual to have lapses in their cognition. Emotional stress can compromise an elder's cognitive status. Victims of elder abuse or individuals involved in stressful litigation may be at risk for stress-induced confusion.

Role of collateral information

Family or other informants may be essential for the evaluation process. They may either be important sources of collateral information or conversely, be potential perpetrators or have some sort of other secondary involvement or gain. This is particularly true for financial exploitation, elder abuse questions, or for potential heirs in a testamentary capacity evaluation Lichtenberg et al., 2015.

Collateral information from direct informants plays an important role in forensic evaluations, particularly with questions of cognitive impairment and dementia. In clinical settings, clinicians who treat older adults often trust collateral sources and take information at face value. However, forensic evaluators must be more objective when it comes to collateral information. Such sources may have a conflict of interest (Kohutis, 2016). This is particularly true in cases of elder abuse and elder financial exploitation, which unfortunately are most often perpetrated by the victim's own family members, and which often means the primary caregiver.

Involvement with families over many years continues into old age. These relationships may be positive or complex and conflicting. Older people are often very involved with their families and not cut off from them.

Review of nursing home and medical records, as well as other documents related to the litigation at hand, is often necessary for a comprehensive forensic evaluation. A comprehensive forensic psychology textbook gives more detailed information on collecting and applying third-party information (Heilbrun et al., 2003).

Physical aging, medical problems, and frailty

Medical problems related to aging can provide essential information in terms of geriatric forensic evaluations. Psychiatric, medical, and neurological records should be reviewed in detail, ideally prior to the interview if possible. The evaluating clinician should consider the results of medical and neurological examinations, laboratory evaluation, brain imaging, and neuropsychological testing (Kohutis, 2016). In addition, substance abuse disorders are projected to increase up to 70% in the elderly baby boomer generation (Rosner, 2017).

As a general rule of thumb: In older individuals, new onset psychiatric symptoms have a physical cause until proven otherwise (Thakur 2015).

Frailty is a complex health state of increased vulnerability, associated with adverse outcomes such as disability, falls, hospitalization, and death. In addition to the reduced physical capacity, frailty might affect selective components of cognition and quality of life. These dimensions should be investigated as part of the forensic assessment process for older adults (Langlois et al., 2012).

Frailty criteria

2 out of 5: pre-frail stage, high risk of progressing to frailty.

3 + out of 5: frailty stage.

Frailty is defined as:

- Low grip strength
- Low energy
- Slowed walking speed
- Low physical activity
- Unintentional weight loss

Fried et al., 2001

Medications and polypharmacy

Older adults are also more vulnerable to the adverse effects of medications. Unfortunately, they are also more likely to be prescribed multiple medications concurrently alongside over-the-counter medications and other supplements.

Prescribing cascade

This can develop when an adverse drug reaction occurs that may be interpreted as a new symptom or illness, resulting in prescribing a new medication. An example is addition of an anti-cholinergic medication for antipsychotic for iatrogenic Parkinson's symptoms.

In some cases, elders are victims of a prescription cascade, i.e. an adverse drug event that is misinterpreted as a medical symptom or condition and results in a prescription for another drug. (Holzer et al., 2018) (Kohutis, 2016).

The Beers Criteria from the American Geriatrics Society (AGS) identifies potential culprits for medications causing adverse effects in older people. In particular, medications, especially with anticholinergic side effects, can affect cognition (AGS, 2015).

Beers criteria (AGS, 2015)

- Used to assess inappropriate medication prescribing the elderly
- Used to identify medications which should be avoided
- Used to avoid medications that are inappropriate with certain medical conditions
- Identifies medications that should be used with caution
- Benzodiazepines, opioids, and anticholinergic medications are especially problematic for cognitive problems and falls

The 3 Ds: depression, delirium, dementia

Geriatric forensic evaluators should be mindful of three common causes for mental health symptoms:

Dementia – chronic cognitive problems, a variety of causes

Delirium – acute confusion caused by a physiological problem

Depression – mood disturbance, symptoms may be different in older adults

By the time the majority of older adults get to a forensic interview situation, their physical, mental, and emotional state have usually been compromised to some degree. When interviewing older adults, clinicians should think of three common causes of mental health symptoms that might be encountered, referred to as the three Ds: dementia, delirium, and depression. As interviewers, it's important to be able to recognize these symptoms.

As a general clinical role of thumb, major depression and/or delirium should be identified prior to considering a dementia-like disorder. Common elements include dysphoric mood, apathy, and forgetfulness. In addition, medical problems, such as vitamin deficiencies, thyroid conditions, and adverse effects of drug therapies can cause all 3 of the D's.

Selected conditions underlying the medical etiology for cognitive deficits reversible

- Hypothyroidism
- Vitamin B12 deficiency
- Central nervous system (CNS) disorders such as normal pressure hydrocephalus (NPH)
- Infections such as syphilis and HIV

First rule out depression and/or delirium prior to considering dementia.

Clinically, the comprehensive initial exam is similar at the beginning of the evaluation irrespective of which of the three D's is being considered. (Scharre and Trzepacz, 2013). An alternative concept is the 6 Ds: Delirium, Drugs, Diseases, Disrupted sleep, Depression, and Dementia. (Wang et al., 2017). All of these can be considered on the differential diagnosis spectrum. Clinicians should carefully review possible differential dementia possibilities.

Routine testing if delirium is suspected

- Thorough physical exam
- Metabolic panel
- Urinalysis
- Urine drug screen

There are many types of dementia. Overall, the importance of dementia in the field of forensic psychiatry cannot be exaggerated. Any physician can diagnose dementia. There is a small role for imaging and biomarkers, but most biomarkers of Alzheimer disease (AD) are invasive, expensive, and difficult to obtain in clinical settings. At this time, neuroimaging is not a diagnostic tool for dementia. The diagnosis of dementia is still primarily based on clinical criteria. (Scharre and Trzepacz, 2013).

Certain disorders (Dementia and Alzheimer's Disease) are much more common in older people. Dementia probably occurs in 8% of those over 65 and 34% of those over 85 years of age.

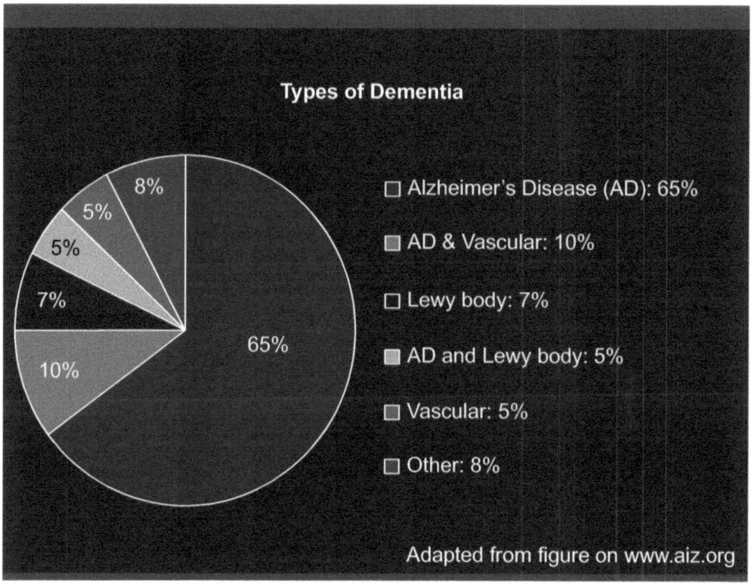

Psychiatric conditions in older adults

Psychiatric problems often present differently in geriatric patients, compared to general adult patients. Typically, geriatric psychopathology develops in the context of medical and neurological disorders. Under these circumstances, ascertainment of symptoms and signs is difficult. Moreover, behavioral abnormalities, cognitive deficits, as well as physical symptoms and signs are often contributed by more than one psychiatric, neurological, or medical condition. Finally, symptoms change over time as various coexisting disease processes progress or subside, which further complicate clinical assessment and diagnosis (Alexopoulos, 2003). Several textbooks discuss these syndromes in detail (Agronin and Maletta, 2011).

Other psychiatric conditions in older adults

This section summarizes some common features of psychiatric conditions in older adults, including 1. Depression, one of the most common psychiatric conditions clinicians will encounter in geriatric forensic evaluations, and 2. Other psychiatric conditions, including psychosis, substance use disorders, and others.

Psychiatric disorders (other than dementia) are probably not more common in older people.

Common psychiatric conditions which affect decision-making

- Substance abuse disorders
- Delirium
- Mood disorders
- Psychosis
- Mild and Major neurocognitive disorders

Like acute cognitive changes, new onset psychosis in an older person should generally be assumed to have a medical cause until proven otherwise. However, if medical causes are ruled out, consider the 6 Ds of psychiatric diagnoses in older adults that co-occur with psychosis and their most likely associated time frame.

The 6 D's of psychiatric diagnoses in older adults that co-occur with psychosis

- Delirium: days to weeks
- Drugs: days to months
- Disease: days to months
- Depression: weeks to months
- Dementia: months to years

Depression

Depression and anxiety in later life, if left untreated, can have far-reaching consequences for an older person. Both can affect executive function (Miller and Reynolds, 2012). Patients with late-life depression have significant impairment in executive functioning. Timely identification of attentional and executive processes is fundamental to the daily functioning of depressed older adults and may require compensation strategies that will improve the outcomes of late-life depression (Lockwood et al., 2002).

Evaluators should not assume that it is "normal" and "understandable" for older people to be depressed. Depression is treatable and should be identified so that it can be treated.

Depression due to a medical condition is not uncommon in the geriatric age group. A disruption in mood is the most salient characteristic of depression. Fewer older adults than younger adults suffer from diagnosable depression. Any abrupt change of functioning should trigger assessment for underlying general medical conditions.

Medical conditions associated with depression in older people

- Alzheimer's disease
- Cancer
- Cardiovascular disease
- Chronic renal disease
- Endocrine disorders such as thyroid disorders
- Infections
- Metabolic disorders
- Neurological diseases
- Parkinson's disease
- Remit illogical diseases
- Cerebrovascular pathology, or stroke

Major depression in older people is often accompanied by a cognitive impairment that spans multiple cognitive domains. MCI emerging during episodes of major late-life depression does not seem to progress to dementia in most cases. However, a history of depression is a risk factor that doubles the likelihood of developing dementia in late life. In the majority of patients, pharmacologic treatment does not lead to major improvement in cognition.

The term pseudo-dementia refers to cognitive deficits that mimic dementia and are due to another condition, usually a psychiatric disorder. There is an increased risk of depression if there is structural brain disease like Alzheimer's or Parkinson's. In addition, a depressed older patient has increased the risk of developing dementia.

Evaluating an older person with depression

- Person should be able to repeat what you have said without any difficulty
- Speech will sound flat; person will appear uninterested, detached
- Listen for indicators of hopelessness, helplessness
- Typical responses include "I don't know" or "I don't care"
- Resignation

Gibson, 2017

Many older adults will have both cognitive and somatic symptoms, which is different from their younger counterparts. They may attribute their symptoms to physical aches and pains or the aging process. An older adult may also have memory complaints due to depression. They may say things like, "I just can't do what I used to do anymore," or "I just can't seem to plan the way I used to plan," or "I think other people are much better off than I am," or "I have a lot more memory problems than most people." (Gibson, 2017).

Somatic symptoms of depression include fatigue or sleep disruption, and either insomnia or hypersomnia. Older adults are less likely to report a depressed mood. Instead, they're more likely to report a lack of purpose, feelings of being burdensome to others or not sure why they are living. They will talk about their sleep disturbances, which aren't uncommon with age, but there is also psychological disturbance, or psychological reasons, as well as physiological causes for sleep disturbance. Therefore, it's important to ask some clarifying questions about sleep disturbance to discover if it's related to mood or dysfunction.

It is known that older adults are at greater risk for completed suicide. The highest risk group for completed suicide is older white males, and seniors make fewer attempts but have a higher rate of successful suicide due to more lethal methods of ending one's life. It's important to listen for passive suicide thinking or death wishes. If a person says, "You know, I am just tired. I'm 92 years old, and I'm ready for God to take me" or if they're denying medical attention. It's important to really understand that, appreciate it, and dig a little deeper in our interview process.

Some of the ways to assess depression are if the person in your interview is able to repeat what you've said without any difficulty. Their speech may sound flat. The person will probably appear very uninterested, detached. Listen for the indicators of hopelessness and helplessness, and some typical responses may be, "I don't know. I don't care," and a sense of resignation that they've given up.

Other psychiatric conditions in older adults

Psychosis

The schizophrenic spectrum and other psychotic disorders in older people are divided according to: [1] early-onset psychosis extending into the patient's old age, [2] late onset psychosis without an.

Underlying medical or logical causation, and [3] late-onset cycles associated with an underlying medical or neurological etiology. The clinician should ask if the illness is early onset with recurrent or chronic history such as schizophrenia, or the new onset of a disorder in later life. The clinician should question if there is a possible medical etiology for the psychosis. Never equate any psychosis at the time of a criminal act with insanity. Brain conditions and neurological syndromes may be associated with the development of psychosis. Schizophrenia likely increases the risk of developing dementia later in life (Holzer et al., 2018).

Active psychosis from schizophrenia can be a problem in criminal, civil, or administrative judicial proceedings. The disease can affect competency of any type and criminal responsibility. Neuro-imaging, particularly an MRI can be obtained as part of the forensic assessment. Those who are violent often demonstrate anatomical brain abnormalities. A neuropsychological assessment for decisional capacity can also be helpful; i.e. the Iowa gambling task (Holzer et al., 2018). Impaired insight into illness is a prevalent feature of schizophrenia and appears to improve modestly during midlife, but then worsen again in later life (Gerretsen et al., 2014).

Intellectual disability

Individuals with intellectual disability are now living much longer with the majority of these people are reaching middle or even old age. The cognitive diagnostic criteria for older people with intellectual disabilities do not provide a clinically useful consensus. Fragile X syndrome, Down syndrome, Prader-Willi and others are at more risk for functional decline, probably to premature aging processes. People with lifelong intellectual disabilities or other neuro-developmental disorders who reach an older age will require cognitive assessment by neuropsychological testing as well as neuroimaging. They may have a lack of capacity due to notable mental developmental impairment, and/or general ability. This is what could be expected in a person with similar impairment when reaching an advanced age (Holzer et al., 2018).

Bipolar disorders

Bipolar and related disorders are separate from depressive disorders. The DSM-5 suggests that bipolar disorders are in between schizophrenia and unipolar depression. Late-onset mania is rare and could be because of medical problems. Unlike major depression, the prevalence of suicide in patients with bipolar disorder tends to decrease with age. Substance abuse is often co-morbid (Holzer et al., 2018).

Anxiety disorders

Anxiety disorders are the most prevalent psychiatric conditions in any age category. Often, the onset of anxiety during old age is due to an underlying medical condition with late onset. Most geriatric patients with anxiety had the onset of the disorder before early adulthood. Anxiety can have a lot of interplay with other issues, including: [1] Alzheimer's, [2] late-onset agoraphobia with a late-life subtype and [3] cognitive impairment. Anxiety symptoms appear to create a cognitive decline in many older adults (Holzer et al., 2018).

Obsessive-compulsive disorders

Obsessive-compulsive disorders have moved from anxiety disorders into their own section. Symptoms of OCD in older adults may be acquired or idiopathic, and related to the dysfunction of frontal-subcortical circuits like Sydenham's chorea, Parkinson's or other dementias. This is an emerging area of research.

Post-traumatic stress disorder

Trauma and stressor-related disorders include PTSD. Women are more likely than men to suffer this condition. Onset may be early or late in life. Victims of elder abuse may be suffering from PTSD.

Hoarding

Hoarding is a common problem among older people and a new diagnosis in DSM-5. Forensic evaluators are likely to encounter older people removed from the home due to hoarding and then having a forensic consultation as a result of unsafe living conditions and an inability to maintain their environment. Based on the current medical evidence, probably all geriatric hoarders should undergo a conference of neuropsychological assessment. Often executive function is impaired, including mental control, working memory, inhibition and set shifting (Holzer et al., 2018).

Substance use disorders

Substance-related and addictive disorders are on the rise in the aging baby boomer population. Older people are more sensitive to the neurotoxic effects of substances, superimposed on age-related changes in the brain. In the coming years, psychiatrists will see greater numbers of substance use disorders and addiction issues in their practices with older adults. Forensic evaluators should be mindful that dual diagnosis disorders, with co-morbid mental illness and substance abuse, produce significant impairment in older people. Excessive alcohol consumption is common among older people. At least 10% abuse alcohol leading to various medical problems. Substance abuse including psychoactive drugs like benzodiazepines can predispose someone to frontal lobe disease (Holzer et al., 2018).

Older adults are less likely to seek treatment or perceive a need for treatment for substance use disorders. However, they may struggle with lifelong substance abuse that continues in older age. They may also develop a substance abuse problem, typically following a major life stressor, such as loss of a spouse, illness, or retirement. Alcohol, prescription medications, and cannabis are commonly abused by older people. These can contribute significantly to cognitive problems.

Mental status examination in older adults

The formal mental status examination (MSE) is the cornerstone of the clinical psychiatric evaluation. A thorough mental status examination is essential for a competent forensic mental health assessment, in order to address both psychiatric and cognitive factors. It allows the clinician to sketch out a more detailed snapshot of the relevant features of the individual examinee. Evaluation techniques are different for the geriatric population than for younger people. In older people, many factors can impact mental functioning and a current mental status examination. These include cognitive factors, sensory deficits including hearing vision and others, the role of co-morbid medical problems, and medications. Both psychiatric and other medications can affect the individuals mental functioning.

The clinician should elicit specific history regarding the specific legal question. This assessment can be critical in a variety of forensic contacts including civil commitment, different forms of capacity, end-of-life decision-making, safe driving, the risk of victimization and abuse, criminal competency and responsibility evaluations, and need for assisted and structured living. Rating scales and tools can augment, but not replace the examination.

Much of the mental status examination relies on indirectly observed data that is assessed continuously throughout the clinician's meeting with the subject. Some aspects of an MSE are diffuse and spread throughout the interview including awareness, speech, thought content, and organization. These include factors like level of awareness and alertness, observation of the fat content, thought process including organization and processing, quality of speech, a state of emotional regulation, behavior, or relatedness. A methodical approach to the mental status exam involves assessment that includes a broad range of areas including [1] behavior, [2] alertness, [3] mood state, [4] thought content and process, [5] sensory input and perception, [6] symptom experience, [7] safety variables, and [8] the different cognitive domains.

The following sections outline key elements of the MSE in older adults, as described in the seminal textbook Geriatric Forensic Psychiatry: Principles and Practice. (Holzer et al., 2018).

Appearance and behavior

The initial presentation and behavior already provide a wealth of data. Outward characteristics include dress, hygiene, posture and gait, motor activity, level of cooperativeness, behavior, and eye contact. Evaluators should consider how to accommodate the interview to make it most effective.

Assessing the degree of cooperativeness and behavior is important. In a forensic context, the subject will normally cooperate, recognizing that it is a serious situation and that their behavior is very important. However, impaired cognition or underlying sociopathy may lead patients to be resistant or act in an agitated or aggressive manner. Excessively friendly or compliant behavior may also signal potential clinical issues from possible misinterpretation of the reason and significance of the evaluation. For example, a criminal defendant with cognitive impairment may be talkative and at risk of self-incrimination (Holzer et al., 2018). Another important behavioral issue is that the elderly may be more vulnerable to the influence of others, which can have forensic implications during a cross-examination.

Possible abnormalities in appearance and affect of an older person

- Restless
- Disheveled
- Suspicious
- Undernourished
- Inattentive
- Confused
- Pale
- Dyspneic

Alertness versus wakefulness

Alertness or wakefulness ranges from a normal range to decreased attention and clouding of consciousness, to lethargy, stupor, and coma. This continuum has been well-described in medical literature and involves the ascending reticular activating system. It is affected by many factors including toxic and metabolic disturbances, drugs, and certain neurological and systemic illnesses. It can adversely affect evaluation and impair the subject's ability to provide a history that is meaningful and to fully participate in an effective examination (Holzer et al., 2018).

Speech and language

Language is fundamental to human communication. Speech and language functioning are distinct and important elements of the mental status exam. A thorough review of language functioning should include assessment of the following: [1] handedness, [2] spontaneous speech, [3] verbal fluency, [4] comprehension, [5] repetition, [6] naming, [7] reading, [8] writing, and [9] spelling. This can be affected by a wide variety of conditions including mechanical problems, such as dysarthria, hypophonia in Parkinson's disease, or drug effects. Poor speech could be because of breathing or hearing changes. Intonation may be unusual or abnormal and this could be a sign of cerebellar disease. A drug-induced state, depression and/or dementia could cause rapid or disorganized speech (Holzer et al., 2018). Dysarthria and stuttering are difficulties in speech enunciation. They should be assessed, but keep in mind they are not necessarily language-based deficits.

Language deficits can have a serious impact in forensic psychiatric contexts. Language problems can affect a subject's communication with law enforcement and attorneys, as well as participation in the evaluation process. The evaluator should make efforts to overcome the deficit and assist the subject to communicate effectively.

Mood

The individual's mood and emotional state are assessed both from the subjective experience of the patient and also by their external expression of emotion. Both of these are important elements of the mental state exam. Many psychiatric, medical, and urological conditions can impact mood and affect. Performance in respect to other aspects of the examination can be affected by impaired mood, state, and/or emotional expression. Mood states range from depression to euphoria. These can be normal reactions or independent from the context or situation. The clinician should consider whether a mood state is appropriate or inappropriate for the context, while also assessing the timing and relationship of emotional reactions to: [1] external factors or precipitants, [2] the degree of fluctuation or constancy, [3] the intensity of the mood state of emotional expression, and [4] whether it is a pure mood state (such as depression or media or a mixed state). Emotional expression through affect can include anger, contempt, disgust, distress, fear, interest, joy, shame, surprise, and/or guilt. The clinician should assess the examinee's emotional expression to determine if it is congruent or incongruent with the stated mood. A disconnection between subjective mood and emotional expression and affect suggests a thought disorder, confusion, a dissociative state, or malingering (Holzer et al., 2018).

Depression can be relevant for forensic implications of abnormal mood states; i.e. if a severely depressed individual admits to a crime he or she did not commit. Apathy is an important consideration in the geriatric population. It refers to a state of indifference, which could reflect either depression or a primary neurological process in the frontal or right hemispheric regions.

Thought content and process

Thought content and quality are continuously assessed throughout the forensic psychiatric evaluation. The clinician may review special areas with the subject, including third-party involvement in non-confidential issues along with a detailed history of illnesses and legal questions or issues related to the case. Various aspects of the fact content are explored throughout the interview. The clinician should pay attention to what the subject reports as being relevant with respect to the context. Is it vague or superficial? Is it over-inclusive and detailed? Either extreme may reflect psychopathology, cognitive disorder, or malingering. Increased feelings of power or creativity may be suggestive of mania. Odd or idiosyncratic content may reflect an underlying psychotic disorder or malingering. The content may include specific areas like thoughts of violence toward self or others (Holzer et al., 2018).

The examinee's thought process describes the rate, flow, direction, association, and connectivity of the patient's thoughts. Generally, healthy thought processing is linear or directional, associated and goal-directed. Pathological fats may be found in: [1] mood and psychotic disorders, [2] cognitive disorders including dementia, [3] medication or illicit drug effects or [4] other active medical and neurological processes. Altered thinking and speech production would present as being too fast or too slow. It is not specific and may signify mood disturbance. Circumstantial thinking is circular and.

Over-inclusive in detail but eventually comes to the point. Conventional thinking is when the subject veers off topic, the endpoint disconnected from the start. Looseness of association and thought is when the speech content is clearly disconnected, and not even obliquely or vaguely connected. Perseveration and viscous thinking are reflected by a subject repeating the fodder topic and unable to shift thinking to a new topic as needed. Thought blocking signifies interruption and thought flow where subject's thoughts get derailed. Neologisms are fabricated words used by subject to communicate thought, though word or words have no definition recognized by others. Word salad is a string of continuous repetitious speech without meaning (Holzer et al., 2018).

Sensory input and perception

Sensory input and perception may show a variety of disturbances associated with underlying psychiatric, neurological, or medical conditions. These could include various sensory modalities like visual, auditory, tactile, olfactory, and/or gustatory. There may be distortions or misperceptions of external or internal stimuli. Misperceptions are distortions that include changes in size, object, shape, intensity, or sound, of stimuli. These could occur in the setting of sensory import disorders, or temporal limbic epilepsy. Hallucinations or other internally created stimuli may occur in various clinical states, including psychosis, dementia, and acute confusion (Holzer et al., 2018).

Lethality assessment

Symptoms and safety assessment could include a survey of the subject experience including: [1] disruptions of sleep, [2] appetite, [3] energy, [4] concentration and attention, [5] interest and motivation and [6] motor functions. Ideas related to thoughts of harm toward self and others should be evaluated, including passive versus active, planning, intensity and how feasible, realistic and achievable the plans are (if present). The clinician should aim to understand the severity of plans with regards to the degree of violence and capacity to be rescued. Impulsivity and concurrent alcohol and drug use should be evaluated. A safety assessment may also include a broader review of the examinee's executive dysfunction, and its impact on personal functioning, such as ambulation and driving (Holzer et al., 2018).

Cognition

Assessments and the degree of detail in the cognitive examination will depend on the legal question at hand, the subject's clinical history, and their deficits displayed during the evaluation. For individuals at higher risk of cognitive impairment (such as in the geriatric population), broad and detailed cognitive evaluation is indicated. If their language appears intact, it may not be necessary to complete a detailed assessment for language separately. A routine psychiatric examination assesses orientation, memory, calculations, language, invite, and judgment. However, when the cognitive domains are divided into more formal spheres of functioning, there are better clinical-pathological and neuro-anatomical correlations. The use of cognitive screening tools may also have a place in certain forensic evaluations (Holzer et al., 2018). These tests are discussed in more detail in Chapter 3.

Memory evaluation is particularly relevant and any disturbance can be due to a wide variety of conditions. In criminal settings, forensic implications of memory assessment are very important since there is a high rate of amnesia claims among defendants. This suggests the importance of valid and standardized procedures for memory assessment. Memory functioning is verbal and nonverbal. The primary process affecting brain regions involved in memory can be responsible for the deficits. Other times, memory deficits can be because of problems with motivation, cooperation, or attention. Stages of memory input include registration and encoding, storage and retention into the longer-term memory, and retrieval of stored information. Memory can be divided into immediate, recent, and remote memory. Immediate memory is a memory trace that can be checked after a few seconds like digit span. Recent memory involves checking daily activities like date, place, and timing, recent news events, and what has happened if a person has had a bad day. Remote memory tests older personal factual information and older historical events like someone's birthday, place of birth, or events that occurred in the past years. It is important that the subject's responses should be verifiable by documentation or by a third-party. A comprehensive test of memory functioning would include immediate recall like digit span, short-term memory like orienting items, long-term memory like personal factual historical information, new learning like word list recall (with and without interference), and visual memory like visual design reproduction.

Visuospatial and constructional abilities involve visual reception, motor functioning, and integration through the parietal brain regions. Areas lying and picture drawings contest this area. This includes copying two-dimensional and three-dimensional drawings and shapes, by asking the subject to draw an object. Visual memory can be tested by repeating a visual task, over time. More complex integrative functions like visual-spatial memory and planning can be assessed. An example of the latter would be having the subject draw a clock and place the hands at a specific time like 10 past 11 (Holzer et al., 2018).

Social cognition is a new cognitive domain described in the DSM-5 and can have some application in geriatric forensic psychiatric assessments. It includes the subject's ability to correctly identify and consider another person's facial emotion and internal emotional or mental state. Some subjects, with specific personality disorders, social dysfunction, sociopath, or brain injury, may have deficits in social cognition. This area could prove very useful in criminal and civil legal contexts.

Higher executive functioning is a somewhat nebulous concept involving the cognitive managerial function to oneself and interactions with the external world. Functions like: [1] planning, [2] reasoning, [3] foresight, [4] moderate monitoring, [5] altering of behaviors, [6] decision-making, and [7] problem-solving are all examples of executive cognitive functions. Intact executive functioning is relatively dependent on other cognitive functions. Impairment in attention, perhaps due to medications, drugs, delirium, or TBI, can adversely affect executive functioning.

Executive functioning tends to be challenging to test. Often the signs and symptoms are observable from the wider evaluation of the patient versus specific techniques in the mental status exam. Practitioners using mental status exams try to approach this area to questions dealing with the fund of information, proverb interpretation abstraction, and an assessment of similarities and differences in items. In general, this area can be assessed throughout the interview by monitoring the subjects' compartment subjectively, by assessing the subject's ability to weigh options, ability to make decisions and plans, ability to inhibit tendencies, reasoning through complex material, and displaying flexibility in thinking, among other capabilities.

Attention

Attention is divided into two categories — simple and complex. Evaluees with significant deficits and attentional functioning may have secondary impairments and other areas of cognition and display limitations in the forensic evaluation. Simple attention is the ability to focus on specific stimuli for a limited period. Digit span forward and backward is the standard test for simple attention. Complex attention involves other variables like the ability to sustain attention over a prolonged period of time, or shift between two different sets of stimuli, or selectively focused attention on a more relevant stimulus and filter out competing but less relevant stimuli. Examples of tests for complex attention would include testing vigilance by asking a subject to respond by tapping every time a specific letter is read.

Rating scales and instruments can be helpful in geriatric forensic psychiatric evaluations. Numerous bedside instruments and scales are available to assist in a mental state examination. They should augment but not replace the in-person mental status evaluation. Examples include scales made to assess global psychiatric symptoms, mood and anxiety, global cognitive functioning, and executive functioning. A standard medical, evidence-based approach should guide the choice of instruments or scales. They should be supported by well-designed studies and references in medical literature. Numerous textbooks review rating scales and instruments that can assist in psychiatric and cognitive mental status exams.

Need for multiple assessments

You may have to complete the assessment over more than one interview to ensure the older person does not become too fatigued to track cognition over time, or in different settings.

Conclusion

Forensic evaluations are different from general psychiatric evaluations. Positive symptom psychiatric disorders and common neuropsychiatric expressions are likely to be seen in geriatric forensic examinees. A traditional psychiatric examination will usually suffice when less clear cognitive or focal neurological signs or symptoms are present.

Selected references

AAPL, 1999. Videotaping of forensic psychiatric evaluations. AAPL task force. American Academy of psychiatry and the law. J. Am. Acad. Psychiatry Law 27 (2), 345–358.

AAPL, 2018. Website of the American Academy for Psychiatry and the Law from. http://www.aapl.org/organization.

Agronin, M.E., 2014. Alzheimer's disease and other dementias : a practical guide. Routledge, Taylor & Francis Group, New York.

Agronin, M.E., Maletta, G.J., 2011. Principles and Practice of Geriatric Psychiatry. Wolters Kluwer Health/Lippincott Williams & Wilkins, Philadelphia.

AGS, A.G.S., 2015. American geriatrics society 2015 updated Beers criteria for potentially inappropriate medication use in older adults. J. Am. Geriatr. Soc. 63 (11), 2227–2246.

Alexopoulos, G.S., 2003. Clinical and biological interactions in affective and cognitive geriatric syndromes. Am. J. Psychiatry 160 (5), 811–814.

American Psychological Association, 2013. Specialty Guidelines for Forensic Psychology.

American Psychological Association, 2014. Guidelines for Psychological Practice with Older Adults.

APA Work Group on Psychiatric Evaluation, Silverman, J.J., Fochtmann, L.J., Vergare, M.J., Anzia, D.J., American Psychiatric Association, 2016. The American Psychiatric Association Practice Guidelines for the Psychiatric Evaluation of Adults. American Psychiatric Association, Arlington, VA.

Buchanan, A., Norko, M.A., 2011. The Psychiatric Report: Principles and Practice of Forensic Writing. Cambridge University Press.

Coste, J.K., 2003. Learning to speak Alzheimer's : a groundbreaking approach for everyone dealing with the disease. Houghton Mifflin, Boston.

Erber, J. a. S., Szuchman, Lenore T., 2014. Great Myths of Aging. Wiley-Blackwell.

Fried, L.P., Tangen, C.M., Walston, J., Newman, A.B., Hirsch, C., Gottdiener, J., Seeman, T., Tracy, R., Kop, W.J., Burke, G., McBurnie, M.A., 2001. Frailty in older adults: evidence for a phenotype. J. Gerontol. A Biol. Sci. Med. Sci. 56 (3), M146–M156.

Gerretsen, P., Plitman, E., Rajji, T.K., Graff-Guerrero, A., 2014. The effects of aging on insight into illness in schizophrenia: a review. Int. J. Geriatr. Psychiatry 29 (11), 1145–1161.

Gibson, S., 2017. Forensic Interviewing with Older Adults. U.S. Department of Justice. Elder Justice Initiative. https://www.justice.gov/elderjustice/video/forensic-interviewing-older- adults.

Glancy, G.D., Ash, P., Bath, E.P., Buchanan, A., Fedoroff, P., Frierson, R.L., Harris, V.L., Hatters Friedman, S.J., Hauser, M.J., Knoll, J., Norko, M., Pinals, D., Price, M., Recupero, P., Scott, C.L., Zonana, H.V., 2015. AAPL practice guideline for the forensic assessment. J. Am. Acad. Psychiat. Law 43 (2 Suppl. l), S3.

Gold, L.H., Vanderpool, D.L., 2013. Clinical Guide to Mental Disability Evaluations, xxv. Springer, New York, p. 394.

Gold, L.H., Anfang, S.A., Drukteinis, A.M., Metzner, J.L., Price, M., Wall, B.W., Wylonis, L., Zonana, H.V., 2008. AAPL practice guideline for the forensic evaluation of psychiatric disability. J. Am. Acad. Psychiat. Law 36 (4), S3–S50.

Heilbrun, K., Warren, J., Picarello, K., 2003. Third party information in forensic assessment. In: Handbook of Psychology.
Heilbrun, K., Grisso, T., Goldstein, A.M., 2009. Foundations of Forensic Mental Health Assessment. Oxford University Press, New York.
Holzer, J.C., Kohn, R., Ellison, J.M., Recupero, P.R., 2018. Geriatric Forensic Psychiatry: Principles and Practice. Oxford University Press, New York, NY.
Janofsky, J.S., Hanson, A., Candilis, P.J., Wade, M., Myers, C., Zonana, Howard, M., Irving, J.B., 2014. AAPL Practice Guideline for forensic psychiatric evaluation of defendants raising the insanity defense. J. Am. Acad. Psychiat. Law 42 (4 Suppl. l), S3–s76.
Kohutis, E.A., 2016. Assessing older adults in civil litigation cases. Int. J. Law Psychiat. 49, 226–232.
Langlois, F., Vu, T.T.M., Kergoat, M.-J., Chassé, K., Dupuis, G., Bherer, L., 2012. The multiple dimensions of frailty: physical capacity, cognition, and quality of life. Int. Psychogeriatr. 24 (9), 1429.
Lichtenberg, P.A., Qualls, S.H., Smyer, M.A., 2015. Competency and decision-making capacity: negotiating health and financial decision making. In: Lichtenberg, P.A., Mast, B.T., et al. (Eds.), APA Handbook of Clinical Geropsychology, Assessment, Treatment, and Issues of Later Life, vol. 2. American Psychological Association, Washington, DC, US, pp. 553–578, 2.
Lockwood, K.A., Alexopoulos, G.S., van Gorp, W.G., 2002. Executive dysfunction in geriatric depression. Am. J. Psychiatry 159 (7), 1119–1126.
Mace, N.L., Rabins, P.V., 2017. The 36-hour day : a family guide to caring for people who have Alzheimer disease, other dementias, and memory loss. Johns Hopkins University Press, Baltimore.
Miller, M.D., Reynolds, C.F., 2012. Depression and Anxiety in Later Life: What Everyone Needs to Know. Johns Hopkins University Press, Baltimore.
Mossman, D., Noffsinger, S.G., Ash, P., Frierson, R.L., Gerbasi, J., Hackett, M., Lewis, C.F., Pinals, D.A., Scott, C.L., Sieg, K.G., Wall, B.W., Zonana, H.V., 2007. AAPL practice guideline for the forensic psychiatric evaluation of competence to stand trial. J. Am. Acad. Psychiat. Law Online 35 (Suppl. 4), S3.
Newlin, C., et al., 2015. Child Forensic Interviewing: Best Practices. U.S. Department of Justice. Office of Juvenile Justice and Delinquency Prevention (OJJDP). Available at: https://www.ojjdp.gov/pubs/248749.pdf.
Pachana, N.A., Laidlaw, K., Knight, B., 2011. Casebook of Clinical Geropsychology: International Perspectives on Practice. Oxford University Press, Oxford; New York.
Reynolds, J., 2016. Case of Elderly Motorist with Dementia.
Rosner, R., 2017. Principles and Practice of Forensic Psychiatry, third ed. Arnold; Distributed in the USA by Oxford University Press, London New York.
Scharre, D.W., Trzepacz, P.T., 2013. Evaluation of cognitive impairment in older adults. Focus 11 (4), 482–500.
Shulman, K., 2018. All about Estates – Blog Posts 2014–2016 from. https://www.allaboutestates.ca/author/kshulman/.
Solie, D., 2004. How to say it to seniors : closing the communication gap with our elders. Prentice Hall Press, New York.
Thakur, M.E., 2015. The American Psychiatric Publishing Textbook of Geriatric Psychiatry. American Psychiatric Pub.
Wall, B.W., 2018. Working with the elderly defendant through the adjudicative process. In: Holzer, J.C., Kohn, R., Ellison, J.M., Recupero, P.R. (Eds.), Geriatric Forensic Psychiatry: Principles and Practice. Oxford University Press, New York, NY.
Wang, S., Nussbaum, A.M., American Psychiatric Association, 2017. DSM-5 Pocket Guide for Elder Mental Health. American Psychiatric Association Publishing, Arlington, Virginia.

CHAPTER TWO

Ethical and legal issues

Contents

An elderly defendant is incarcerated in the county jail. The forensic psychiatrist was asked to conduct an evaluation of competence to stand trial. The defendant has late stage cancer and last used cannabis two days before his incarceration. During the evaluation, he seems confused, glancing around room, oriented to person only responses generally irrelevant to the questions being asked. He nevertheless responds correctly to several questions, knows roles of

The Clinician's Guide to Geriatric Forensic Evaluations
ISBN: 978-0-12-815034-4
https://doi.org/10.1016/B978-0-12-815034-4.00002-7

courtroom personnel, the difference between a felony and a misdemeanor, the concept of pleading guilty or not guilty, and understands what a and plea bargain is.

(Salem and Leonard, 2009).

Ethics in dementia

Clinicians, caregivers, and policy makers face daily challenges in striving for the best quality of life for people with dementia and their family and caregivers. A significant gap exists between the first signs of dementia and an actual diagnosis, often 2–3 years or more. Only about half of the patients with dementia who see their primary care doctor on a regular basis receive a diagnosis (Neuroschl and Welle, 2011).

Ethical and legal issues associated with progression of dementia

- The emergence of preclinical and asymptomatic at-risk categories for dementia creates complex questions about preventive measures, risk disclosure, and protection from stigma and discrimination
- Tmportant research continues to investigate ways to alleviate clinical dementia's symptoms, and requires additional human subjects' protections to ethically enroll persons with dementia
- Changing needs of people who continue to live with dementia

Johnson and Karlawish, 2015

Expanding the boundaries surrounding the concept of dementia to include asymptomatic, but at-risk persons, generates new ethical questions. One promising way to address these questions is to take an integrated approach to dementia ethics, considering the interdisciplinary nature of ethical questions related to dementia including: [1] health policy questions about insurance coverage for long-term care, [2] political questions about voting, [3] driving and [4] other civic rights and privileges as well as [5] economic questions about balancing an employer's right to a safe and productive workforce against an employee's rights to avoid discrimination on the basis of their dementia risk (Johnson and Karlawish, 2015).

An improved understanding of dementia patients' experiences provides a new impetus to address legal and ethical issues. There are many emerging issues in relation to their awareness and impact on legal and ethical matters, which include concepts of: [1] beneficence, [2] non-maleficence, [3] autonomy and [4] paternalism. These concepts can be applied in relation to: [a] advance directives, [b] capacity, [c] decision-making and [d] participation in research and treatment (including informed consent and truth-telling). Tensions exist between the imperatives of doing no harm and of maintaining autonomy in addressing legal and ethical issues (Woods and Pratt, 2005).

The main ethical and legal issues that arise in dementia involve mental competence or the capacity to make personal decisions. Mental competence is task-specific. An incapacity to do one thing does not necessarily imply incapacity to do another. For example, a dementia sufferer may be competent to write a will, but unable to manage his/her financial affairs. Also, because of task specificity, thresholds within types of competence may vary. Competence, like innocence, is presumed. However, on the other hand, incompetence must be established. Status (which includes a diagnosis of a psychiatric condition, dementia or emergency psychiatric detention) does not necessarily confer incompetence. On the other hand, an outcome is not a criterion by which to judge competence. In other words, competent people have the right to make wrong decisions (Jacoby, 2006).

In summary, there are many ethical, legal, medical and forensic issues that are faced by the older adult population with dementia, associated with their care. Most prominent among these issues is the maintenance of autonomy while ensuring their safety and the safety of individuals who care for them. Decisions regarding end-of-life, including the formulation of advance directives, add to the complexity of care for this demographic. A significant portion of individuals in the criminal justice system are aging and many have psychiatric disorders, which are further complicated due to the lack of services (Tampi et al., 2018).

Professional guidelines

It is critical for clinicians to be familiar with the specific requirements and standards in the jurisdictions in which they practice. Physicians must recognize that the best way to avoid legal problems is to be aware of the legal requirements in the jurisdictions in which they practice. Nevertheless, with regards to the provision of clinical services, it is best to think clinically (and not legally) regarding the provision of consistency and in terms of sound clinical care to patients (Brendel et al., 2010).

The American Academy of Psychiatry and the legal ethical guidelines for the practice of forensic psychiatry (Glancy et al., 2015) include the following categories.

1. Preamble: A forensic psychiatrist practices at the intersection of psychiatry and law, with the inherent potential for complications, conflicts, misunderstandings and/or abuses.
2. Confidentiality: This can be a significant problem in a forensic situation. Notice should be given as to any limitations. Precautions should be taken to ensure that none of the confidential information received falls into the hands of any unauthorized person or entity.
3. Consent: This is one of the core values of the ethical practice of medicine and psychiatry. Some situations (such as court-ordered evaluations) do not require consent. In such cases, a psychiatrist should inform the subject that an evaluation is legally required and that even if the subject refuses to participate, the fact will be noted in any report or testimony.
4. Honesty and striving for objectivity: There are hazards, given the adversarial nature of the Anglo-American legal process. There is potential for unintended bias or distortion of the expert's opinion. All data should be considered. Contingency fees are not acceptable.
5. Qualifications: Required expertise is claimed only in areas of actual knowledge and skills, training and experience. Expert qualifications should be presented accurately and precisely.
6. Procedures for handling complaints of ethical conduct

Ethics in forensic evaluations

To the practicing clinician, ethics often seem theoretical and remote from everyday forensic work. However, it is important to remember that geriatric forensic clinicians and evaluators are valuable to the justice system only by virtue of their integrity. The ethics of our field are central to the entire forensic process, including geriatric forensic report writing.

Constructive input from medical experts can help the court, even when there are competing opinions. Ethical practice and decision making in geriatric forensic evaluations require an awareness and understanding of the ethical issues and challenges that are commonly encountered when working with older adults in clinical and forensic contexts.

Although multiple resources are available to assist practitioners in identifying common ethical issues and challenges, experienced colleagues often serve as one of the richest sources of information and recommendations. The experiences and advice of senior colleagues provide an important perspective to help clinicians anticipate, avoid and address ethical challenges (Bush et al., 2015).

Ethical values to consider

The right to self-determination

Ethical goals in psychiatry include promoting personal autonomy and enhancing the protection of people with diminished capacity. In situations where the person is mismanaging or endangering themselves or others, geriatric forensic evaluators must balance the impact on the individual's dignity and their right to make risky decisions with the benefits of protecting that vulnerable individual from potential harm. At times, an individual's right to self-determination, dignity and right to make risky decisions will take priority over the paternalistic need to protect the individual from potential harm.

Professional competence

As an expert, your pertinent knowledge, skill, experience, training, and education can help the court understand the evidence or determine a fact.

In order to qualify as an expert, you must have something special to contribute. Courts have rules about such pre-requisites. The role distinction between an expert witness and a fact witness is outlined in the table below.

Differences between a fact witness/treating expert and a retained expert

	Fact witness/ Treating expert	Retained expert
1. Who is the client?	The patient	Retaining attorney, Court
2. Forms doctor-patient relationship	Yes	No
3. Provides treatment & explains test results	Yes	No
4. Advocates for patient	Yes	No
5. Relies extensively on records and other collateral contacts	Not Necessarily	Yes
6. Services provided within adversarial context	No	Yes
7. Provides forensic opinions on causality & permanency	No	Yes
8. Knowledgeable about facts of legal matters/claims made	Not Necessarily	Yes
9. Fiduciary responsibility to whom?	The patient	Retaining attorney, Court
10. Professional services paid by whom?	The patient and/or insurance company	Retaining attorney, Court

Richards et al., 2015

Some states have adopted a rule requiring that a party needs show that evidence is scientifically valid and reliable. Qualifications may be: [1] academic or operational, [2] local, [3] national, [4] international, [5] general and/or [6] specific. You may be considered an expert because of your background, experience, or knowledge.

Since most cases involve difficult questions, you should showcase your competency in whatever field you offer your services. Attorneys, judges, and juries will evaluate your ability by your public qualifications and items you list on your CV, including: [1] education, [2] training [3] practical experience, [4] professional and technical expertise, [5] position and function and/or [6] recognition by professional associations, awards and/or publications. The trier-of-fact is the jury. In non-jury court trials, the judge is both the trier-of-fact in the trier-of-law.

Qualifying as an expert

- Prior to 1993, most federal courts relied on the 1923 case of Frye v United States, that held that proposed scientific testimony be peer-reviewed, i.e. generally accepted by others in the field.
- In 1993, Daubert v Merrell Dow Pharmaceuticals brought in the rule so that any expert who might help the trier-of-fact may be heard.
- Knowledge, skill, experience, training, or education can help the jury understand the evidence or determine a fact, the expert may testify. The judge can make an assessment of whether or not the testimony's underlying reasoning or methodology is scientifically valid and is applicable.

Forensic versus therapeutic role

The psychiatric expert witness has several roles to play when participating in the legal process, including: [1] consultant, [2] business person, [3] teacher, [4] advocate, [5] witness and [6] performer (Gutheil and Simon, 2002). There are specialized ethical guidelines for forensic psychiatrists. In the setting of forensic psychiatry, the principle of justice is mainly characterized by professionalism, the principle of beneficence by objectivity and impartiality and the principle of respect of autonomy by informed consent, as well as the principle of non-maleficence — defined as the non-collaboration of the psychiatrist in any activity leading to inhuman and degrading treatment or to the death penalty (Niveau, 2018).

Institutionalization and civil commitment

Every clinician and, at least one occasion during professional career will seek to have a patient institutionalized, will be called to testify as a lay or expert witness during civil commitment proceedings.

Additional ethical guidelines in geriatric forensic psychiatry involve basic rights being at stake; i.e. in dementia and guardianship cases. They include: [1] reliance on potentially biased collateral sources (particularly for financial capacity evaluations), [2] reporting/regulatory/public safety issues for occupational and driving capacity and [3] the capacity to marry and sexual consent questions (particularly in nursing home settings).

Importance of self-care

As geriatric forensic professionals, we must also pay attention to our own self-care. Vicarious trauma or compassion fatigue can develop in professionals who do this work, which is shaped by our own prior experiences and our own histories with aging. It's also important to understand our own individual beliefs about autonomy versus protection, our beliefs about aging and any myths that we have. These concepts are shaped not only by our own society and the society of ageism but our own personal experiences. When we are faced with a really challenging case that pushes up against our own values and beliefs, we should consult with our colleagues (Gibson, 2017).

- Self-Reflections
- Importance of self-care
- Prior experiences
- Similarities/differences in child versus Older adult forensic interviewing
- Beliefs about autonomy and protection shaped by society and personal experiences
- Myths or beliefs about aging
- Infantilizing language

Gibson, 2017

Further reading: Ethics in forensic psychiatry

- The Ethical Practice of Forensic Psychology: A Casebook (Pirelli et al., 2016)
- Forensic Psychiatry: Clinical, Legal and Ethical Issues, Second Edition (Gunn and Taylor, 2014)
- Ethical Issues in Forensic Psychiatry: Minimizing Harm (Sadoff, 2011; Appelbaum and Gutheil, 2007; Glancy et al 2015; Bush et al., 2017; Streim, 2015; Reid, 2013)

Integrity and impartiality

Multiple relationships/conflicts of interest

The ever-expanding role of geriatric forensic experts in civil litigation has led to a higher level of expectation in realms such as: [1] clinical and courtroom knowledge, [2] objectivity and [3] work product utility. Geriatric forensic evaluators need to recognize that bias is inherent in clinical and forensic work. It is imperative that in high stakes situations such as forensic geriatric assessment, the evaluator is proactively conscientious in recognizing, and minimizing, the effects of these biases.

Common biases affecting geriatric forensic evaluators during evaluations, as well as during depositions or trial testimony include role, cognitive, and practice biases. Specific suggestions are available from both empirical literature and forensic experience on how to recognize and mitigate such biases (Richards et al., 2015).

12 Sources of bias in forensic neuropsychology

- Role bias: Conflating clinical and forensic roles
- Financial/Payment bias
- Referral source bias (and retaining attorney pressure)
- Self-report bias (Need for corroborative data)
- Under-utilization of base rates
- Ignoring normal variance in test scores
- Confirmation bias
- Personal and political bias
- Group attribution error
- Diagnosis momentum
- Good old days bias
- Overconfidence

Adapted from Richards, 2015

Avoid taking requests directly from litigants

Requests from complainants or litigants themselves, rather than from their lawyers or legal representatives, should almost always be declined. Such people may misunderstand or misrepresent their situations, provide inadequate information to potential experts, and/or not understand the legal or administrative issues in their cases. Any of these issues can create difficulty for the potential expert and they may encourage inappropriate, unethical or even illegal activities (Reid, 2013).

Working with attorneys

Consultation:
A lawyer's conversation with a clinician to discuss concerns about the client's presentation. Usually client is not identified and consultation does not require client consent.

Referral:
A formal referral to a clinician for evaluation, which may or may not result in a written report. Requires client consent.

ABA/APA, 2008, p. 121

Lawyers play an important role in protecting the interests of vulnerable older adults. Ethical principles prohibit lawyers acting on anything other than (legally) competent instructions, and disapprove of acting 'in the best interests' of clients in the absence of competent instructions.

What information do you need from the lawyer?

Background information about the client and the circumstances;
The reason for referral - the legal issue at hand; and.
The relevant legal standard.

ABA/ABA, 2008, p. 123

It is important to establish a formal business relationship with the retaining attorney to clarify who is hiring you and what you are being hired for. Before testifying, you should do research, read documents and give opinions. Late calls from attorneys shortly before trial can place an undue burden on the experts, (Reid, 2013).

When and why a lawyer might seek your help

- Determination of whether a prospective client has sufficient legal capacity to enter into a lawyer-client relationship;
- Determination of whether a client has capacity to undertake a specific legal transaction;
- Evidence in a guardianship proceeding;

When and why a lawyer might seek your help (*cont'd*)

- Expert testimony in a deposition or courtroom hearing;
- Clarification of the areas of diminished capacity, as well as retained strengths;
  - Affirmation of the client's capacity;
- Expert opinion on conclusions of other psychological evaluations, including those submitted by opposing counsel;
  - Justification of the attorney's concerns about capacity to disbelieving clients and family members;
- Expert advice on strategies to compensate for identified mental deficits;
- Indication of the need for protective action by the attorney; and
- Recommendations concerning any follow-up testing.

ABA/APA, 2008, p. 121

Negotiating schedules can be a difficult calculation. You have to balance the time necessary to review cases against possible reports, depositions and trials. Long dormant cases may suddenly erupt into action. Case-related activities may occupy your time for indefinite periods of time. The rhythm of the legal system may involve continuances, postponements and uncertainties of trial scheduling and duration. Planning for depositions, preparing and rehearsing testimony and clarifying the specific role function of the experts are elements of preparation with retaining counsel. Experts should manage these complexities and help arrive at solutions that are ethically sound and useful to the legal system (Gutheil and Simon, 2002).

Fees and financial relationships

Business aspects of forensic work include managing fee agreements and finances in a forensic practice. Attorneys and courts are the major sources of forensic income for private practitioners. The practice of contingency fees, contingent on the successful outcome of the case, are ethically barred since the practice is thought to contaminate the objectivity of the expert's opinion and to link the expert inappropriately to the case outcome. The threat of nonpayment for a divergent opinion is an inappropriate for an expert witness.

The use of fee agreements is customary and may include retainer agreements, based on the estimation of anticipated time and costs. Clear and stable fee policies make for good business boundaries. Topics may include retainers and advance payments, standard fees versus different fees for different services, day rates, travel and practical aspects of good expert practice (Reid, 2013).

Legal issues

A legal primer

American law is broadly divided into four areas:

- Constitutional **law** sets the basic framework for governmental powers, civil rights, and civil liberties.
- **Statutes** are enacted by elected legislatures, and set out provisions that may be quite broad in scope or fairly detailed.
- **Administrative rules**, regulations, and policies, interpret and flesh out the statutes.
- **Case law** is the body of principles and rules arising from specific disputes heard in the courts. Judges apply constitutional, statutory, and administrative law to individual conflicts, as well as the principles derived from previous cases, to resolve cases and controversies.

Court decisions provide guidance in interpreting and applying existing law to the real world, while sometimes creating new law. The aggregate of reported cases on a particular subject form a body of jurisprudence referred to as *common law* doctrine. According to the principle of *stare decisis*, courts adhere to decided cases or "precedent" unless the court finds a compelling reason to overrule it, thus creating new precedent.

When lawyers and judges use the term "legal standard" for capacity, they mean he definition or test of capacity as it exists in statutory law as interpreted by any existing administrative guidelines and case law. For instance, a statutory definition of "testamentary capacity" may be clarified by will contests in court. A definition of "incapacity" in guardianship law may be translated into practical terms by a court's evaluation form.

Statutes are written at the local, state, and federal levels. For most capacities in this book, and for adult guardianship, the relevant laws are at the state level. State courts that address matters of civil capacity or guardianship may be specialized family or probate courts, or they may be courts of general jurisdiction in which a judge may be less familiar with the particular issues at stake.

ABA/APA, 2008, p. 16

Geriatric criminal evaluations

Increase in number and percentage of arrests

- Inmates aged 55 + is the fastest growing group of prisoners
- Growing at six times the overall growth rate
- People aged 65 + who are given prison sentences increased 63% from 2007 to 2010, while the general population increased by only 0.7% in the same period
- It is projected that growth rates of this age group being incarcerated will continue to rise (Yarnell et al., 2017)

Dementia and crime

Because of the high rates of dementia found in older first-time offenders, many experts recommend that a thorough cognitive evaluation should be conducted on all older adults who enter the legal system (Yarnell et al., 2017). Of first-time offenders aged 60 + who were referred for forensic psychiatry evaluation, it is estimated that more than 50% of them have been diagnosed with a psychiatric disorder. The most common diagnosis is dementia (Yarnell et al., 2017).

Elderly defendants constitute a heterogeneous group of first-time offenders, as well as repeat offenders. Charges can vary widely in the degree of severity. Most elderly criminals serving sentences are in prison for violent offenses, and they are often repeat offenders. However, the elderly mostly commit property crimes such as shoplifting. Factors that may help explain first-time offenses by the elderly include marital and family issues, such as: [1] the loss of loved ones or the emergence of spousal abuse, [2] alcohol and drug use, [3] cognitive impairment, [4] increased aggression and [4] uninhibited sexual behavior (which may constitute symptoms associated with neuro-cognitive disorders). Non-prescription use of prescription medications among the elderly has been an emerging public health concern. Most elderly people who use illicit substances began using them before age 30, and clinical referral in later life often stems from legal charges (Holzer et al., 2018).

Geriatric forensic psychiatrists have an important role after sentencing, as well. Studies have shown that some inmates with advanced dementia are unable to recall their crimes or even to understand why they were incarcerated in the first place. Although reminded of their crimes before a parole hearing, they may not even remember their offenses and, therefore, are incapable of showing remorse. Thus, the possibility of parole is significantly limited. Ergo, the fairness of a parole denial at such a hearing is questionable. In these situations, geriatrically-informed treatment or forensic psychiatrists could review an individual's case to help determine an appropriate outcome and placement. These providers could also help ensure that appropriate medical and behavioral techniques are used in the treatment of such inmates (Yarnell et al., 2017).

Sociopathy in older adults

The elderly are not often thought of as being associated with criminal activity. Epidemiological studies on antisocial personality disorder and FBI crime statistics provide an understanding of sociopathy and directed aggression in the geriatric population. Acts that may be considered to be criminal are usually carried out by individuals with major neuro-cognitive disorders, particularly, fronto-temporal neuro-cognitive disorder (Holzer et al., 2018).

Though not often studied in the elderly and not yet studied using DSM-5 criteria, antisocial personality disorder (ASPD) as defined by DSM-IV criteria is found in a small proportion of the aged population. According to estimates from the National Epidemiological Survey on Alcohol and Related Conditions (NESARC), the rate of ASPD in the elderly population (age <65) is 0.6%, compared to 6.2% for the group 18–29 years, 4.2% for ages 30–44, and 2.8% for ages 45–64. Age 65 + years was associated with a significantly decreased risk of ASPD (odds ratio 0.09) compared to the reference ages of 18–29. Rates of ASPD are higher among substance abusers; however, this is only partially true in the elderly population. Among elderly persons who met criteria for any lifetime DSM-IV alcohol use disorder: [1] rates of ASPD increased to 2.4% total, [2] with 2.9% among males and 0.95% among females. However, among elderly persons with a history of any lifetime DSM-IV drug use disorder, the rates of ASPD remained low, at 0.3% total — respectively 0.4% for males and 0.0% for females (Holzer et al., 2018).

Malingering/feigning

Two reports from the 1990s suggest that at least 10% of defendants who are referred for competency evaluations attempted to feign mental problems that would impair competence. Judges consistently cite malingering as a reason for their skepticism about the defendants' having genuine mental disorders (Janofsky et al., 2014). Occasionally, forensic clinicians encounter referrals for competency evaluations that seem frivolous because the defendant is obviously competent. However, clinicians should recognize that when a defendant displays signs of a competence-impairing mental disorder, the defense counsel is obligated to question whether the client can proceed with adjudication (Janofsky et al., 2014). It was ruled in court, though, that difficulty in ascertaining whether a defendant is incompetent or malingering may make it appropriate to place the burden of proof on them, but it does not justify the additional onus of an especially high standard of proof (Glancy et al., 2015).

Because of the severe consequences of a defendant's malingering, psychiatrists should not make this diagnosis lightly. Solid evidence, not clinical suspicion, should be the basis of such a diagnosis (Janofsky et al., 2014).

Potential sources of confirmatory evidence of malingering

- Psychological testing or specialized instruments for detecting malingering
- Medical, psychological and/or custodial records
- Interviews with family, friends, police, custodial officers and others who have had contact with the defendant
- History with the criminal justice system

Janofsky et al., 2014

When interviewing the defendant, the evaluator will look for inconsistencies in the story, medical history, observed behavior and previous assessments. If the psychiatrist suspects malingering but he/she does not have sufficient evidence to make that diagnosis, he/she can recommend that the defendant enter an inpatient unit, where around-the-clock observation can help confirm or deny the charge of malingering (Glancy et al., 2015).

Adjudicative process

Working with the elderly defendant through the adjudicative process presents many challenges. Views vary on the degree of discretion that law enforcement, judges, and juries should grant in the adjudication and sentencing of elderly defendants. There has been a growing number of elderly defendants and a sharp rise in elderly offenders and elderly adjudications.

Elements of the adjudicative process

- Detention, Booking, and Initial Hearings
- Mental Competency to Stand Trial
- Physical Competency to Stand Trial
- Discovery and Trial
- Disposition and Appeal

Holzer et al., 2018

Older people have a higher chance of diminished cognitive functions and this can hinder the entire legal process. For example, it is important that the defendant fully understands the charges brought against him/her and are able to assist the attorney in his or her own defense. The attorneys, judge, and forensic psychiatrists should all be sensitive to the fact that elderly defendants may need more frequent competency evaluations (Holzer et al., 2018).

It may be necessary to make accommodations for elderly defendants during the process of adjudication, such as: [1] competency to stand trial, [2] physical competency and [3] other medico-legal issues, which may require expert medical and mental health involvement. Elderly offenders with cognitive or physical impairments, particularly those that contributed to the commission of the criminal act, may not fully deserve the criminal punishment meted out to non-elderly offenders. In many cases, it seems appropriate to consider age as a mitigating factor, especially when physical and mental health are also relevant to sentencing.

According to a 2002 report, the types of competency deficits seen in the elderly differ from those found in younger defendants. The deficits of younger defendants are attributable to functional psychiatric illness rather than the organic decline of impairment seen in older offenders (Frierson et al., 2002). The same report studied competent and incompetent defendants and found that while the median ages were similar between the two groups, one significant difference between the two was the existence of dementia. 19% of competent defendants were diagnosed with dementia, whereas 90% of incompetent defendants had dementia (Frierson et al., 2002).

Being familiar with neuropsychiatric issues, consulting with other disciplines such as neurology, and ruling out treatable causes of neuro-cognitive disorders are important elements of conducting competency assessments in this population (Glancy et al., 2015). When beginning a criminal competency assessment, it is important to establish the defendant's global level of functioning and his/her specific knowledge and understanding regarding the pending proceedings (Kirkish and Sreenivasan, 1999).

Steps to conduct forensic assessments for criminal proceedings

- Prepare for the interview
- Provide notice
- Obtain background information
- Mental status examination
- Questions specific to adjudicative competence
- Elicit the defendant's account of events that led to the charge
- Psychological testing

Glancy et al., 2015

Competency to stand trial

Competency means that the defendant can consult with his/her lawyer and can factually and rationally understand the legal proceedings at hand. CST evaluations of elderly defendants require preparation. Before the assessment, the forensic evaluator must obtain police records (incident reports, witness statements, crime scene reports, autopsy reports, etc.) in order to facilitate assessment of the defendant's ability to understand the legal charges and relevant evidence in the case. The defendant's medical records, including past medical, psychiatric, and jail treatment records, should also be gathered. These may reveal mental health diagnoses or medical concerns, which may potentially impair a defendant's CST. While an older person's medical records may be extensive, the focus should be placed on records documenting recent functioning, since a CST evaluation concerns present-state functioning. Jail records may also contain information about the defendant's functioning in the jail environment and the presence of behavioral disturbances, while incarcerated, that may recur in the courtroom setting (Holzer et al., 2018).

Ethically, the evaluator should ensure that the defendant has been appointed counsel and that counsel is aware of the evaluation. The examiner should also inform the defendant about the nature and purpose of the evaluation, the agency of the evaluator (court appointed or retained by defense or prosecution) and the limitations of confidentiality.

If cognitive impairment or other symptoms interfere with an elderly defendant's capacity to understand this information, the defendant's counsel should be made aware of it and an offer to be present during the interview should be made. Additionally, if a defendant presents with cognitive deficits, obtaining collateral information from a spouse, family members or jail personnel, may provide information about the duration, previous medical workup, and impact of such deficits on the defendant's daily functioning. The degree of cognitive impairment seen in major neuro-cognitive disorders, especially in Alzheimer's disease, can manifest more prominently later in the day. This is also true for delirium, since disturbances in attention and awareness may fluctuate over time. If an attorney reports that an elderly client appears to have trouble understanding information related to his legal case, but a CST evaluation does not reveal an explanation for such difficulty, the evaluator may wish to assess the defendant over several occasions at different times during the day. A person evaluated for CST may perform very well during a morning evaluation but poorly later in the day. Because criminal trials can last many days (or even weeks in some jurisdictions), an inability to maintain consistent cognitive functioning and follow trial process throughout an entire day may warrant either an opinion of a lack of CST or a recommendation for abbreviated trial days (Holzer et al., 2018, p. 164, p. 164).

In virtually all jurisdictions, a defendant may be compelled to undergo a mental health evaluation as a prelude to a hearing regarding his/her competence to stand trial. Such evaluations may compromise a defendant's fifth amendment protection against self-incrimination because they may admit to certain actions either spontaneously, or in response to the psychiatrist's questions (Glancy et al., 2015).

Evaluating clinicians are given minimal guidance concerning what level of capacity justifies a finding of competence. In stating that the defendant must have 'sufficient present ability' to work with his attorney, the legal system leaves it to the trial court to decide whether a defendant's abilities suffice for a finding of adjudicative competence (Glancy et al., 2015). The evaluating psychiatrist needs to give the defendant enough time, and needs to interview with enough thoroughness, in order to make a thorough assessment of the functional characteristics, which are relevant to the jurisdiction's legal criteria for adjudicative competence. If reasonable attempts to examine the defendant fail because of a lack of cooperation or other factors, then he/she should report such limitations to the referral source. Poor performance, or lack of participation, are not, by themselves, determinative of incapacity. In cases in which the psychiatrist anticipates that language barriers, religious beliefs, sensory impairments (e.g., hearing impairments) or other communication factors will create impediments to accurate assessments.

If there is a language barrier, the geriatric forensic evaluator should arrange (with the prior agreement of the referring attorney or court) to use interpreters or other individuals who can facilitate communication. And, of course, the interview should always be conducted in a secure location.

The primary purpose of a competency evaluation is neither diagnosis nor treatment. The goal of the evaluation is to evaluate whether mental symptoms exist, and if so, how they impair competence-related abilities. It is important that the defendant know that the evaluation process differs from ordinary doctor-client confidentiality. For this reason, the defendant's normal physician should not be the evaluator in legal proceedings.

Components of competency to stand trial (CST)

- Does the defendant know with what he/she is charged with?
- Does the defendant know who is representing him/her and his/her role in the court process?
- Does the defendant understand the trial process and the roles of the other participants in it?
- Does the defendant appreciate the consequences of his/her trial?
- Is the defendant able to cooperate and collaborate with his/her representative?

The relevance of severe symptoms in regards to the question of competence varies from case to case. Nevertheless, it is still valuable to obtain enough information about a defendant's condition in order to identify diagnoses that are relevant to the expert's opinion. In cases in which the psychiatrist believes that the defendant lacks adjudicative competence, diagnostic information will provide valuable information regarding the defendant's restorability and the proper setting for restoration (Glancy et al., 2015). In addition, the results of an evaluation of the defendant help the court, including the judge and jury, to get closer to the truth even though it won't always help the defendant.

There are no universal certification requirements for forensic evaluations during court proceedings, but some states are moving toward required certification of forensic expertise for those conducting such assessments. Recent data indicate inconsistencies in the application of the existing standards even among forensic experts. However, the recent publication of consensus guidelines may foster improvements in this arena. There are also ongoing efforts to develop and validate structured instruments to aid in competency evaluations. Telemedicine-based competency interviews may facilitate evaluations by those with specific expertise for the evaluation of complex cases. There is also interest in the empirical development of educational methods to enhance adjudicative competence.

The attention of the courts (and, implicitly, the attention of the psychiatrist) is directed to the defendant's 'ability' to consult rationally with an attorney, rather than the defendant's willingness to consult rationally. The term 'reasonable' connotes flexibility in determining competence, while the phrase 'rational as well as factual understanding' requires the courts and psychiatrists to consider broadly how the defendant exercises his cognitive abilities (Glancy et al., 2015).

Components of capacity to assist counsel

- Understanding of criminal charges
- Understanding of the implications of being a defendant
- Understanding of the adversarial nature of the proceedings
- Understanding the role of defense counsel, the prosecutor, the judge and the jury
- Ability to work with an attorney and relate pertinent information
- Ability to make important decisions that arise during adjudication (how to plead, how to consider plea deals, defense strategy, etc.)

In evaluating claims of amnesia, the psychiatrist should consider the purported genesis of the memory deficit and collateral information (e.g., hospital records or reliable witness statements from the time surrounding the alleged offense) in attempting to determine the plausibility and authenticity of the amnesia. Medical records may also provide the psychiatrist with data that help determine whether the defendant's presenting symptoms are compatible with his/her medical history. Findings from psychological testing (including assessments of malingering) may also help the psychiatrist to evaluate a defendant's assertions about amnesia. Psychiatrists are trained to offer an opinion on the matter, following a clinical examination which should include a review of the relevant past and present history and mental state. Psychologists often apply one of many specific testing instruments designed to answer the same questions. There is no evidence to suggest that one approach is superior to the other. In studies which compare the outcome of psychiatric versus Psychological opinions on this matter, there is no significant difference.

Tools for competency to stand trial evaluation

- MCGARRY CAI TOOL: a competency assessment instrument that assesses 13 areas of functioning as it relates to trial competency
- MACARTHUR CST TOOL: a competency screening tool that assesses financial capacity and the capacity to consent to medical treatment

With regard to competency evaluations, the IQ itself may lend data to support the opinion that a defendant lacks capacities associated with competence to stand trial. The most common reason that defendants are deemed incompetent is their inability to form a collaborative relationship with an attorney to assist in their own defense. This capability is difficult to measure. Although the quality of the patient's relationship with mental health professionals often serves as a proxy for the defendant's capacity to formulate collaborative, working relationships with others, the nuances of the attorney-defendant relationship differ from those of the therapeutic relationship, and are not always apparent.

Restoration of competency to stand trial in older adults

Restoration of competency refers to the process of a defendant regaining the competency required to continue with the legal process. After an incompetent determination has been made, most statutes explicitly require that the psychiatrist formulate an opinion about whether the restoration of competence is likely within some statutorily designated time frame, which is usually linked to the severity of the potential penalty for an alleged crime (Glancy et al., 2015). If restoration appears likely, psychiatrists in some jurisdictions must also render an opinion about the range of services that will be necessary to restore the defendant to competence (Glancy et al., 2015). Competency restoration options include psychiatric hospitals, outpatient programs and jail-based programs. The options available to defendants depend on the jurisdiction.

Evaluators are encouraged to assume that defendants' competencies can be restored, except in cases of irreversible impediments such as mental retardation and progressive dementia. Defendants with dementia are not likely to have competency restored because it cannot be treated or reversed.

Considerations for the probability of competency to stand trial restoration

- Whether the defendant's incompetence results from a treatable deficit, such as a lack of prior exposure to information about the trial process or psychiatric symptoms caused by an illness that typically responds to medication as opposed to a static and relatively irremediable condition such as intellectual disability
- The defendant's previous psychiatric treatment and responses to treatment
- The character of presenting symptoms and current scientific knowledge about how well those symptoms respond to treatment
- The fact that research on competence restoration shows that most individuals referred for treatment after being found incompetent do become competent to stand trial

Glancy et al., 2015

Older defendants were less likely to be restored and successfully adjudicated. The typical non-restorable defendant had slightly lower level charges — meaning that he/she was diagnosed with [1] a psychotic illness, [2] low cognitive functioning, [3] both a psychotic illness and low cognitive functioning, or [4] was prescribed more medications and had a history of prior episodes of incompetence. Regardless of the timeframe for competence efforts, psychiatrists should recognize, however, that courts may regard a "low" but >0 probability of success to be "substantial" enough to warrant a trial of restoration.

Articles on the adjudicative competence of older defendants generally find that deficits in orientation and memory best distinguish competent from incompetent older defendants. Advanced age and a dementia diagnosis are associated with non-restorability. Increased age correlates with non-restorability, even after correcting for a dementia diagnosis (Glancy et al., 2015).

Insanity defense

Courts have repeatedly made a distinction between findings, regarding fitness for trial and criminal responsibility (which is related to a defendant's mental state when the alleged offense took place). These are independent determinations on distinct ultimate issues. A finding that a defendant is competent to stand trial cannot prevent him from trying to establish an insanity defense, and such a finding is not admissible at trial (Janofsky et al., 2014).

Forensic psychiatrists, in addition to evaluating competency, conduct assessments to evaluate insanity defenses (AAPL). Ongoing cases have continued to refine the definition of insanity, and each state has specific evaluations to determine sanity in a case. Insanity defenses are rare. In the U.S., they represent <1% of felony trials and are successful <25% of the time and only 7% of the time in jury trials.

Evaluation criteria for insanity defense

A criminal defendant in federal court is incompetent to stand trial if a preponderance of the evidence shows that he 'is presently suffering from a mental disease or defect, rendering him mentally incompetent to the extent that he is unable to understand the nature and consequences of the proceedings against him or to assist properly in his defense' (Glancy et al., 2015). Competency is equivalent to the defendant's current ability to understand. On the other hand, sanity refers to the defendant's mental state at the time the crime was committed.

Severity of mental illness for an insanity plea

In many jurisdictions, insanity statutes require the presence of a severe mental disorder. They exclude diagnoses of non-severe mental disorders, though these may still be permissible bases for findings of incompetence to stand trial.

While the U.S. Supreme Court does not regard the insanity plea as a constitutional right that states must make available to defendants, a criminal defendant has a constitutional right to be tried only when competent (Glancy et al., 2015). When a defendant is found not guilty by reason of insanity, the defendant does not typically walk free. Rather, the inmate undergoes treatment or institutionalization, as required by that state.

Presentencing evaluations

Most forensic evaluations are ordered to determine whether a person's psychiatric illness interferes with their ability to perform a task; i.e. to stand trial, to control conduct or understand wrongfulness. In contrast, presentencing evaluations are performed to determine whether a convicted defendant is a fit subject for punishment. There is significant jurisdictional variation in the use of presentencing evaluations. They can provide a judge the opportunity to consider a variety of factors when deciding a sentence. In the federal system, the judge can consider information about a defendant's past criminal record, his/her assistance to law enforcement, as well as, other factors that could call for an upward or downward departure from standard sentence recommendations (Holzer et al., 2018, p. 167).

Older offenders in correctional settings

The demographics of the prison system are changing. The effects of dementia on the accused, the incarcerated and the prison system in general are palpable.

There currently is no consensus regarding what age to use in designating an offender as "older." Varying studies have grouped older offenders in the range of 50–70 with the majority beginning to classify older offenders at 55+. The Bureau of Justice Statistics has recommended age 55 as the beginning age range for "older offenders." The primary reason for this recommendation is that it's related to the differentiation made between an older offender's physiological and chronological age. An incarcerated offender's physiological age can be 10–15 years older than their chronological age. Risk factors present prior to and during incarceration are responsible for this discrepancy. Pre-incarceration risk factors for accelerated aging include: [1] inadequate access to preventative medical care, [2] substance abuse, [3] poor diet, [4] stress, [5] lower socioeconomic status and [6] a history of previous incarcerations. Post-incarceration correctional environmental risk factors include: [1] high-fat and high-carbohydrate diets, [2] stress, [3] being vulnerable to victimization, [4] social isolation and [5] physical inactivity. 55 + offenders exhibit poorer overall health status with higher rates of chronic physical illness, mental illness and functional impairments, than younger offenders or older community-based comparison groups (Holzer et al., 2018).

Chronological age is not always the best tool to measure expected functionality and healthcare needs. A younger offender with a head injury might exhibit more cognitive and functional deficits than a 65-year-old with good overall general health. Therefore, in addition to chronological age, a measurement of functional ability that is specific to the needs and challenges of older adults in correctional settings would help identify target groups and support the delivery of adequate healthcare to this population.

Differing terminology exists for offenders regardless of their age. Within adult correctional settings, the terminology is typically based on current legal status, legal definitions, or location (jail, detention center, etc.). State or federal offenders are typically referred to as inmates or offenders. We refer to the older jail detainee, state or federal prisoner or other correctional or institutional setting inmate, as an "offender" or "offender patient." Research has identified three categories of older adult offenders: [1] first-time offenders, [2] recidivists and [3] long-term servers. First-time offenders are individuals who have committed their first crime after the age of 50. Their crimes tend to be more serious and receive longer sentences. These offenders are likely to have more difficulty adjusting to the stress of incarceration and are more vulnerable to stress-related health conditions. Recidivists are habitual offenders who have experienced multiple incarcerations at various ages that are associated with new sentences or parole violations. Recidivists tend to exhibit more health issues related to substance abuse and chronic health conditions related to the lack of healthcare access. Long-term servers are offenders with long sentences, who have aged in the correctional setting. This demographic of offenders is typically not prone to acute stress-related health issues but they experience more chronic conditions (Holzer et al., 2018).

This classification system of older adult offenders requires further development and elaboration. This includes linkage with offender patient-specific medical and mental health treatment programs, targeted to address their needs, in order to minimize healthcare costs and improve their quality of care. Prisoners have a constitutional right to timely access to care for their serious medical needs.

Correctional healthcare systems are facing the challenge of providing adequate and cost-effective care for the ever-increasing older demographic with chronic medical conditions, such as diabetes, cardiovascular disease, end-stage liver disease, cognitive impairments and/or mental illness. Older offenders have special medical needs that sometimes present with psychiatric symptoms of depression, delirium, acute psychosis and/or other behavioral issues.

Factors supporting adequate health care for older offenders

- Use of a consistent definition of older offender
- Use of a consistent definition of functional impairment in the correctional setting
- Improved correctional and medical staff training in the specific needs of older adults
- Recognition and assessment of dementia and mental illness

(Continued)

Factors supporting adequate health care for older offenders (*cont'd*)

- Establishment of geriatric housing units
- Adapting existing prison facilities to accommodate functional impairments
- The development of re-entry plans that target the specific needs of older adults upon release
- Early medical release programs.

Holzer et al., 2018

Selected references

American Bar Association and American Psychiatric Association, 2008. Assessment of Older Adults with Diminished Capacity: A Handbook for Psychologists. ABA/APA, Washington, DC.

Appelbaum, P.S., Gutheil, T.G., 2007. Clinical Handbook of Psychiatry & the Law. Wolters Kluwer/Lippincott Williams & Wilkins, Philadelphia.

Brendel, R.W., Wei, M.H., Schouten, R., Edersheim, J.G., 2010. An approach to selected legal issues: confidentiality, mandatory reporting, abuse and neglect, informed consent, capacity decisions, boundary issues, and malpractice claims. Med. Clin. 94 (6), 1229–1240.

Bush, S.S., Allen, R.S., Molinari, V.A., 2017. Ethical issues and decision making in geropsychology. Ethical Prac. Geropsychol. 22.

Bush, S., Allen, R., Heck, A., Moye, J., 2015. Ethical issues in geropsychology: clinical and forensic perspectives. Psychol. Injury Law 8 (4), 348–356.

Frierson, R.L., Shea, S.J., Shea, M.E., 2002. Competence-to-stand-trial evaluations of geriatric defendants. J. Am. Acad. Psychiatry Law 30 (2), 252–256.

Gibson, S. 2017, Forensic Interviewing with Older Adults. (2017) U.S. Department of Justice, Elder Justice Initiative https://www.justice.gov/elderjustice/video/forensic-interviewing-older-adults

Glancy, G.D., Ash, P., Bath, E.P., Buchanan, A., Fedoroff, P., Frierson, R.L., Harris, V.L., Hatters Friedman, S.J., Hauser, M.J., Knoll, J., Norko, M., Pinals, D., Price, M., Recupero, P., Scott, C.L., Zonana, H.V., 2015. AAPL practice guideline for the forensic assessment. J. Am. Acad. Psychiat. Law 43 (2 Suppl. l), S3.

Gunn, J., Taylor, P., 2014. Forensic Psychiatry: Clinical, Legal and Ethical Issues, second ed. CRC Press.

Gutheil, T.G., Simon, R.I., 2002. Mastering Forensic Psychiatric Practice: Advanced Strategies for Expert Witness. American Psychiatric Publishing, Inc, Arlington, VA, US.

Holzer, J.C., Kohn, R., Ellison, J.M., Recupero, P.R., 2018. Geriatric Forensic Psychiatry: Principles and Practice. Oxford University Press, New York, NY.

Jacoby, 2006. Ethical and Legal Issues in Dementia. Ethical and Legal. Elsevier.

Janofsky, J.S., et al., 2014. AAPL practice guideline for forensic psychiatric evaluation of defendants raising the insanity defense. J. Am. Acad. Psychiat. Law 42, S3–S76.

Johnson, R.A., Karlawish, J., 2015. A review of ethical issues in dementia. Int. Psychogeriatr. 27 (10), 1635–1647.

Kirkish, P., Sreenivasan, S., 1999. Neuropsychological assessment of competency to stand trial evaluations: a practical conceptual model. J. Am. Acad. Psychiat. Law 27 (1), 101.

Neugroschl, J., Wang, S., 2011. Alzheimer's disease: diagnosis and treatment across the spectrum of disease severity. Mt. Sinai J. Med. NY 78 (4), 596–612.
Niveau, G., Welle, I., 2018. Forensic psychiatry, one subspecialty with two ethics? A systematic review. BMC Med. Ethics 19 (1), 25-25.
Pirelli, G., Beattey, R.A., Zapf, P.A., 2016. The Ethical Practice of Forensic Psychology: A Casebook. Oxford University Press. Incorporated.
Reid, W.H., 2013. Developing a Forensic Practice: Operations and Ethics for Experts. Routledge.
Richards, P., Geiger, J., Tussey, C., 2015. The dirty dozen: 12 sources of bias in forensic Neuropsychology with ways to mitigate. Psychol. Injury Law 8 (4), 265–280.
Sadoff, R.L., 2011. Ethical Issues in Forensic Psychiatry: Minimizing Harm. Wiley.
Salem, A., Leonard, C., 2009. Psychiatric and clinical sequelae of delirium and competence to stand trial. J. Am. Acad. Psychiatry Law 37 (4), 549–551.
Streim, J.E., 2015. In: Sadoff, R.L. (Ed.), Forensic Issues in Geriatric Psychiatry. Oxford University Press, New York, pp. 155–162.
Tampi, R.R., Young, J., Balachandran, S., Dasarathy, D., Tampi, D., 2018. Ethical, legal and forensic issues in geriatric psychiatry. Curr. Psychiatr. Rep. 20 (1), 1.
Woods, B., Pratt, R., 2005. Awareness in dementia: ethical and legal issues in relation to people with dementia. Aging Ment. Health 9 (5), 423–429.
Yarnell, S.C., Kirwin, P.D., Zonana, H.V., 2017. Geriatrics and the legal system. J. Am. Acad. Psychiat. Law 45 (2), 208.

CHAPTER THREE

Evaluation of cognitive impairment

Contents

The Clinician's Guide to Geriatric Forensic Evaluations
ISBN: 978-0-12-815034-4
https://doi.org/10.1016/B978-0-12-815034-4.00003-9

Cognitive changes in older adults

Normal aging

Cognitive and mental disorders are **not** part of normal aging. Physiological changes in aging affect all systems, including metabolism. Metabolism affects how the person handles medications and environmental stressors. In older people, medications and polypharmacy are common causes of confusion.

There is a cognitive continuum among older adults of "super aging" (describing people in their 70s and 80s who have the mental or physical capability of their decades-younger counterparts), normal aging, mild cognitive impairment (MCI), and dementia. Cognitive performance over the lifespan falls into 2 key categories: crystallized intelligence (learned knowledge) rises into a person's 60s, but fluid intelligence to solve flexibly and novel problems declines from age 20 (Weintraub, 2017).

The line between what is considered age-appropriate memory change and age-inappropriate change is blurry. Overall, the effects of normal aging on cognitive function and memory are quite modest and are seldom brought to clinical attention. Nonetheless, the context of aging and the common fear of dementia among many older individuals sometimes lead to great concern over occasional memory lapses, whimsically referred to as "senior moments".

Normal aging or dementia?

Age-appropriate versus age-inappropriate cognitive change

- Normal aging is associated with some deterioration in memory, attention, and processing speed and accuracy
- There may be an overall decline in short-term (or immediate) memory which is not related to a progressive dementia

Normal aging or dementia? (*cont'd*)

- Older subjects actually perform better on some memory tests, an effect that may be attributed to increased overall knowledge
- Heterogeneous pathways of cognitive aging are an emerging area of research

Agronin (2014); Price (2013)

Normal cognitive aging can mean a decreased ability to think fast and synthesize, starting around age 53.

Older adults undergo these changes around the same time they are facing complex financial challenges, at age 65 and beyond, simply as a part of normal aging. These include retirement, higher fixed costs and increased funds needed for expenses, relocation, refinance of mortgage, estate plan, business succession, assets protection, charitable plans, long-term health care, nursing home, desire to maintain autonomy etc. Generational changes mean an increasing proportion of older adults are helping their adult children with down payments, loans or education expenses.

Many older adults undergoing normal aging may actually become more optimistic as they age, increasingly seeing the world through rose-colored glasses. The downside of this is that elders may lose healthy suspicion for untrustworthy individuals and be more susceptible to scams. It is important to note that this can be a part of normal aging, and is not necessarily due to underlying pathology of the Alzheimer's type or other dementia processes (Boyle, 2012; Han, 2016b). Even normal cognitive aging can impair an older person's ability to make complex financial judgments and to resist undue influence.

Changes in executive functioning

It is well established that executive function plays a pivotal role in cognition, but there is no consensual definition yet. Executive function is an umbrella term for a wide range of higher-order cognitive processes that coordinate a person's skills needed for planning, initiation, and control of complex, independent, appropriate and purposeful goal-directed behavior. Executive function refers to a complex set of processes that manage and control other functions. It is one of the most important domains of decision making.

Executive functions are like the "CEO" of the brain and they control purposeful, goal-directed behaviors. Like the CEO of a company, the brain's executive function system continuously monitors and directs the brain's organizing and regulating "departments" so it can proceed as effectively and efficiently as possible. Neuroanatomically, the executive function system is situated in the frontal lobes, cortical and subcortical structures.

What is executive function?

Executive function includes cognitive, emotional, and motor abilities, including the ability to self-monitor, plan, organize, reason, be mentally flexible, and problem-solve. It guides how people organize their lives, plan, and implement their plans.

Executive function deficits

Damage to the executive function system can lead to:

- Difficulty with organizing, planning, and initiation
- Unawareness or denial that their behavior is problematic
- Inability to multitask
- Difficulty processing, storing, and retrieving information
- Difficulty with verbal fluency and understanding abstract concepts
- Inability to learn from consequences of actions
- Loss of interest in activities
- Socially inappropriate behavior including lack of concern for people and animals

Executive function skills generally decline even with normal aging. What happens when executive function is impaired? Since the brain's executive function system organizes and regulates information across numerous cognitive domains, impairment in executive function typically involves multiple deficits. Loss of higher level "administrative" guidance and control can cause behavioral change. Furthermore, profound executive function deficits can lead to serious problems in safety, function, employment, and emotional well-being.

In normal aging, a person can experience a decline in concept formation, abstraction, and mental flexibility, especially after age 70. There can also be a normal age-related decline in response inhibition (the ability to inhibit an automatic response in favor of producing a spontaneous new response), reasoning with unfamiliar material, and executive abilities requiring a timed motor component.

Many of the central questions in geriatric forensic psychiatry are governed by questions of an individual's executive functioning, particularly the capacity for decision making. Executive function is also critical for an individual's ability to live interpedently, be aware and protect oneself, and behave according to societal norms. It is needed to meet the demands of everyday life in a flexible and adaptive manner. It is strongly correlated with a person's functional abilities.

Everyday activities affected by executive function disturbances

- Medical and financial decision-making
- Instrumental activities of daily living
- Housework
- Hygiene
- Transportation
- Shopping
- Meal planning

Holzer et al., 2018

Executive function can be impaired, even when other basic cognitive functions are relatively preserved.

Forensic psychiatrists performing evaluations of older adults should remember to assess executive function.

Several relatively brief bedside assessments of the executive function are available. A few of these are discussed later in this chapter. In some cases, it may be best to undertake a comprehensive neuropsychological assessment of the executive function in consultation with a neuropsychologist.

Common neuropsychological tests for executive function, with norms for older individuals up to at least age 80

- Trail Making Test A and B
- Delis Kaplan Tests of Executive Function
- Wisconsin Card Sorting Test
- Category Test

(Continued)

Common neuropsychological tests for executive function, with norms for older individuals up to at least age 80 (*cont'd*)

- Stroop test
- Verbal fluency tests

Holzer et al., 2018

In younger individuals, attention deficit hyperactivity disorder (ADHD), mania or substance abuse may be common causes of impaired executive function. Depression or delirium is less common. For some individuals, many factors could have been involved, however age-related changes or subtle onset of dementia should be considered, even in the absence of gross deficits in dimensional cognitive testing such as in a Mini Mental State Examination (MMSE), which notoriously fails to properly assess executive function parameters.

Red flag for early dementia: poor decisions about money

An important indicator of early Alzheimer's disease is when people begin to make bad decisions regarding money. If an older adult suddenly changes and gives a lot more money to telemarketers or new "friends", that's a red flag. Incipient dementia may well be at work.

Importance of decision-making abilities

Decision making is a complex executive function that draws on past experience, present goals, and anticipation of outcome. It is influenced by emotions and culture. For the functional neuroanatomy of decision-making, a large brain circuitry is involved. Interactions between the free prefrontal regions are described in the previous image with subcortical structures. The more complex the decision, probably the more all of this circuitry is at play (Rosenbloom et al., 2012).

Brain circuitry in decision making

- Frontal cortex
- Prefrontal regions
- Limbic system
- Basal ganglia

Brain circuitry in decision making (*cont'd*)

- Thalamus
- Cerebellum
- Pons

Currently, data is very limited regarding the effects of early neuropsychiatric changes on the domains such as medical decision-making, consenting to medical research studies, engage in legal contracts, financial decisions, driving, composing a last will and testament etc. It can also affect complex decision-making, for example reporting facts to the dispatcher on a 911 call.

Decision-making that may be affected by MCI or early dementia

The ability to:

- Respond to emergencies
- Pilot or drive transportation vehicles
- Make medical decisions and manage complex medical treatments
- Stand trial, testify as a witness, qualify as a juror
- Handle firearms
- Fulfill social and occupational roles
- Engage in intimate sexual relations
- Recognize fraud or scams
- Resist undue influence over personal decisions
- Manage finances
- Execute a will and last testament

Decision-making is defined as a complex executive function that draws on past experience, present goals, anticipation of outcome, which is influenced by prevailing and predicted emotional tone and cultural context (Rosenbloom et al., 2012). The decision-making process depends upon interactions between the three prefrontal regions described in the previous image with subcortical structures that include the limbic system, basal ganglia, thalamus, cerebellum, and even the pons, which is part of the brain stem. It is a vast circuitry.

There are many complex decision-making capacities that may be affected by early Alzheimer's disease or mild cognitive impairment. Decision-making in the context of mild cognitive impairment, say as a part of early Alzheimer's disease, is a precarious situation. An individual may well be at risk regarding their ability to make financial decisions and their ability to thwart undue influence (See Chapter 5 for more in-depth discussion of elder financial exploitation, elder abuse and undue influence.).

Medical and legal frameworks for evaluating and determining the capacity to perform these life activities vary greatly among specific tasks from state to state. There are few agreed-upon medical or legal guidelines. No reliable instruments are available to measure susceptibility to undue influence and coercion. Adequate data is lacking regarding the effects of early neuropsychiatric changes on domain of functioning such as medical decision-making consenting to medical research studies, engaging in legal contracts, making financial decisions, voting, operating a motor vehicle, and composing a last will and testament (Edersheim et al., 2017).

Family members, legal authorities, and healthcare providers may erroneously conclude that intact judgment is present inadequate performance on passive orientation, memory and calculations. It's interesting how family members and healthcare providers actually overestimate capacity in most people, especially if the older person agrees with the recommendations that are being made by the medical treatment team or by the family.

Mild cognitive impairment (MCI)

Mild cognitive impairment (MCI) refers to subtle cognitive decline, where activities of daily living remain unimpaired, with an estimated 10% −15% yearly conversion rate toward Alzheimer or other type of dementias. Neurochemistry, structure, and clinical impact all come together in a progressive, nuanced gradual insidious process ending in dementia. Mild cognitive impairment (MCI) is considered an intermediate stage between normal aging and dementia. It is diagnosed in the presence of subjective cognitive decline and objective cognitive impairment without significant functional impairment, although there are no standard operationalizations for each of these criteria.

Behavioral and cognitive correlates in MCI

- Impaired Awareness
- Depression (20%), apathy (15%), irritability (15%)
- Diminished complex decision-making capacities including medical and financial decisions
- Increased risk of motor vehicle accidents

Price 2013

What is dementia?

The term dementia literally means "without a mind" in Latin. Although dementia is still the most commonly used diagnostic term, revisions in the diagnostic nomenclature have replaced it with neurocognitive disorder. For now, the term dementia continues to be widely used and understood, is familiar to readers across medical specialties.

Definition of dementia

- Loss of memory and other mental abilities severe enough to interfere with daily life, caused by physical changes in the brain
- Acquired, generalized and usually progressive impairment of cognitive functions including memory, orientation, and language that does not affect level of consciousness
- Progressive cognitive decline of sufficient magnitude to interfere with normal social or occupational functions, or with usual daily activities
- Memory may not necessarily be impaired in the early stage but is usually affected eventually
- Attention, executive function, and visuo-perceptual ability may be affected instead of memory

Age is the biggest risk factor for dementia. The prevalence of dementia doubles every five years after age 65. There is a great diversity of subtypes of dementia, each with its distinct features. Mixed dementias are very common, more likely the norm. Diagnosis is mostly clinical, with the gold standard being autopsy postmortem. The Text Box below presents general ways to classify the dementias. Increasingly, these boundaries are seen as fluid, since most dementias contain elements of both categories. Nevertheless, such classifications have been broadly used. Regarding biomarkers, 30%—40% have a positive biomarker, but it is unclear if they actually lead to Alzheimer's disease or what their relevance is.

Ways to classify dementia

- Reversible (arrestable/modifiable, e.g. hydrocephalus, TBI, infections) versus Irreversible (e.g. Alzheimer's disease)
- Progressive (e.g. Alzheimer's, Creutzfeldt-Jakob) versus Non-progressive (e.g. TBI, certain strokes)
- Cortical (e.g. Alzheimer's) versus Subcortical (e.g. Parkinson's dementia)

Agronin 2014

How common is dementia?

Today, 10 million Americans suffer from dementia. Alzheimer's disease accounts for about half, with mixed presentations being very common. In 2050, 19 million people will have Alzheimer's disease, not counting other dementias. In the United States alone, rates of Alzheimer's disease (AD) is at epidemic proportions, afflicting approximately 5.4 million individuals, with 96 % being older than 65. Of this older group, 63 % are female (Alzheimer's Association).

The main risk factor for all forms of dementia is age, and with the number of older Americans projected to nearly double in the next 30 years, there will clearly be a tremendous surge in the number of dementia cases, barring any major advance in prevention or treatment. It is estimated that AD and other dementias afflict over 35 million people worldwide currently, with a projected increase of over 155 million people by 2050 (Alzheimer's Association). Most of the increase will take place in developing countries, including China and India.

The annual cost of treating dementia in the United States was estimated to be between $157 billion and $215 billion in 2010, eclipsing the costs of both heart disease and cancer. Dementia and Alzheimer's are leading causes of death, which are not usually listed on death certificates.

Symptoms of dementia

Common dementia symptoms

- Memory Loss
- Confusion
- Disorientation (advanced)
- Language problems
- Inability to recognize familiar objects
- Changes in personality or behavior
- Disturbance in executive functioning

Behavioral neurological disorders such as dementia often require a brain-based assessment (in addition to the classical psychiatric emotion-based assessment) as part of a forensic psychiatric examination. Overlap may exist in symptoms and deficits in some psychiatric and neurological disorders. A forensic psychiatrist may need to organize consultations with neuropsychologists, neuroradiologists, laboratory pathologists, and other specialists to complete the comprehensive forensic geriatric psychiatric evaluation.

The last FDA approved medication for Alzheimer's disease was released in 2003. Around 400 clinical trials were conducted over the past 15 years with a nearly 100% failure rate. Over 100 medications were tested in clinical trials, but it remains unclear if they have any effect.

Dementia versus Alzheimer's disease

Many patients and caregivers confuse the terms dementia and Alzheimer's disease. One simple way to educate them is to explain that dementia is a general term, like infection, and there are different types. If a doctor told you that you had an infection, a natural question would be "What type of infection do I have?". Remember that everyone who suffers from Alzheimer's disease has dementia, but not everyone with dementia has Alzheimer's disease (Agronin, 2014).

Challenges in diagnosis

There is generally a delay in symptoms, often 2–4 years, prior to formal diagnosis of Alzheimer's disease, because this is an insidious process, progressing slowly over the years (Granacher, 2018). Many factors come together to minimize the impact including intact social graces, intact personality structure, preservation of most ADLs, overestimation of one's own cognitive skills, masking behaviors congruent behaviors, accepting as normal aging, denial, fear, therapeutic nihilism by family friends and doctors since there is no cure and no highly effective disease altering treatment. Denial of the dementing process is common in affected patients and their families and communities.

Different systems for diagnosing dementia

There are multiple systems for diagnosing dementia and its various types. Later in this chapter we will take a closer look at the current version of the American Psychiatric Association Diagnostic and Statistical Manual (DSM-5), the most relevant classification for psychiatrists, despite the 2013 introduction of new and somewhat unwieldy terminology unique to psychiatry and psychology, used to describe the dementias. Beyond the DSM, two other major classification systems are the ICD and the AA/NIA criteria for Alzheimer's.

Beyond the DSM: other systems for diagnosing dementia

- 11th Revision of the International Classification of Diseases (ICD-11)
- Alzheimer's Association (AA) and the National Institute on Aging (NIA) – only for Alzheimer's dementia

The International Classification of Diseases (ICD) is the international "standard diagnostic tool for epidemiology, health management and clinical purposes". The ICD is revised periodically and is currently in its 10th revision. ICD-10, as it is therefore known, is from 1992 and the WHO publishes annual minor updates and triennial major updates. The World Health Organization is currently revising the International Classification of Diseases (ICD) toward the ICD-11.

The Alzheimer's Association and the National Institute on Aging (NIA), an agency of the U.S. National Institutes of Health (NIH), jointly issued four new criteria and guidelines in 2011 to diagnose Alzheimer's disease. By incorporating new scientific insights and technological advances, the new guidelines aim to improve current diagnosis, strengthen autopsy reporting of Alzheimer's brain changes, and establish a research agenda for future progress in earlier detection and even greater diagnostic accuracy. Three of the new guidelines focus on three stages of Alzheimer's disease: (1) dementia due to Alzheimer's, (2) mild cognitive impairment (MCI) due to Alzheimer's, and (3) preclinical (pre-symptomatic) Alzheimer's. The fourth guideline updates criteria for documenting and reporting Alzheimer's-related changes observed during an autopsy. (https://www.alz.org/research/diagnostic_criteria/).

The NIA/AA diagnostic guidelines for Alzheimer's disease (AD) were designed to reflect recent research which indicates that AD begins affecting the brain many years before problems in memory, thinking, and learning are noticeable. This means that if we can develop ways to detect and treat the disease in the pre-symptomatic stage, we can prevent symptoms occurring, i.e. prevent dementia (Jack, 2018).

Multidisciplinary treatment of dementia

Dementia is frequently managed by clinicians in multiple disciplines. For many subtypes, multidisciplinary international expert groups have developed specialized consensus criteria based on clinicopathological correlation with underlying brain pathology.

Neurobehavioral /neuropsychiatric symptoms of dementia

Neuropsychiatric symptoms in cognitive impairment mainly include the so-called behavioral and psychological symptoms of dementia, or BPSD. These are symptoms of disturbed perception, thought content, mood or behavior that frequently occur in patients with dementia, a heterogeneous array of symptoms, signs, and syndromes. BPSD are present in up to 97 % of clinical situations, including community and nursing-home populations. These symptoms are responsible for premature institutionalizations, huge direct and indirect costs, and above all considerable suffering and diminished quality of life on the part of people with dementia and their families (Verdelho and Gonçalves-Pereira, 2016).

Neuropsychiatric, behavioral and psychological symptoms of dementia (BPSD)

- Behavioral: wandering, agitation/aggression, resistiveness to care, inappropriate sexual behaviors, catastrophic reactions, sundowning
- Psychological: psychosis—delusions, hallucinations—misidentification, depression, anxiety, apathy

Verdelho and Gonçalves-Pereira (2016)

Evidence for distinct neuropsychiatric behavioral features in NCDs has been recognized, as well as neuropsychiatric symptoms of dementia or BPSD (behavioral and psychological symptoms of dementia), particularly in the areas of psychotic symptoms and depression. Individuals with NCD can present with a wide variety of behavioral symptoms that are the focus of treatment. Psychotic features are common in many NCDs, particularly at the mild-to-moderate stage of major NCDs, due to Alzheimer's disease, Lewy body disease, and frontotemporal lobar degeneration. The Text Box below lists common neuropsychiatric symptoms clinicians may find associated with DSM-5 Neurocognitive Disorders.

Neuropsychiatric behavior disturbances of dementia

- **Mood disturbances**, including depression, anxiety, and elation, may occur. Depression is common early in the course. Mood symptoms are a significant feature in the earliest stages of mild NCDs such that clinical recognition and intervention may be important.

(Continued)

Neuropsychiatric behavior disturbances of dementia (*cont'd*)

- **Paranoia and other delusions** are common features and often a persecutory theme may be a prominent aspect of delusional ideation.
- **Agitation** is common in a wide variety of NCDs, particularly in major NCD of moderate to severe severity, and often occurs in the setting of confusion or frustration. It may arise as combative behaviors, particularly in the context of resisting caregiving duties such as bathing and dressing.
- **Sleep disturbance** is a common symptom that can create a need for clinical attention and may include symptoms of insomnia, hypersomnia, and circadian rhythm disturbances.
- **Apathy** is reflected in diminished motivation and reduced goal-directed behavior accompanied by decreased emotional responsiveness
- **Hallucinations**
- **Other behaviors**: wandering, disinhibition, hyperphagia, and hoarding

Holzer et al., 2018

Neuropsychiatric symptoms of dementia:

Amnesia

The term amnesia denotes an impairment of memory. Memory consists of a diverse set of psychological processes and brain systems involved in learning and retrieving information. It is often divided into working memory, declarative memory (episodic and semantic), and nondeclarative memory (implicit and procedural).

Types of memory

- Working memory
- Declarative (factual)
- Nondeclarative

"Amnesia" is used often to describe impairments in declarative (factual) memory, particularly new learning memory. It can be anterograde (inability to form new memories subsequently to the event that produces the amnesia), retrograde (inability to recall information acquired before the event that produced the amnesia), or both anterograde/retrograde (global amnesia).

Types of amnesia

- Anterograde (inability to form new memories)
- Retrograde (inability to recall previously acquired information)
- Both

When examining patients with memory deficits, a forensic evaluator should describe the type of the memory impairment associated findings in neurological, mental status, or neuropsychological testing. The generic term amnesia is relatively vague and should be avoided unless more detail is given.

Clinicians should be aware that family members and healthcare providers may overestimate capacity in many older people. Family members, legal authorities and healthcare providers may erroneously conclude that intact judgment is present from adequate performance on passive orientation, memory and calculations (Price, 2013, Holzer et al., 2018).

Apathy

Many individuals with early Alzheimer's disease or other dementias have apathy, i.e. diminished motivation, social withdrawal, passivity, and difficulties with task completion. Apathy is prominent in early and advancing Alzheimer's disease, including the pre-symptomatic, prodromal, and later clinically apparent dementia. It may appear to be a personality change or depression.

Apathy is associated with lower motivation, lower persistence, decreased concentration, social withdrawal, and disengagement. These are all neuropsychiatric symptoms which have a huge impact on complex decision-making, for example in a context of being cognizant of undue influence, and ward against fraud. Even in early Alzheimer's disease these alterations take place.

In addition, early dementia, particularly Alzheimer's disease, also often involves increase in associated neuropsychiatric symptoms of anxiety, depression, and agitation. Combine that with the lack of insight awareness concern, and their usual overestimation of their cognitive abilities, and you can see that a perfect storm is beginning to form for individuals with early dementia (Price, 2013).

A Norwegian study of a naturalistic population (Bruen et al., 2008) showed apathy is prominent in early probable Alzheimer's, and that 74%, even in early Alzheimer's disease, have apathy.

Agnosias

Agnosia, or "not knowing", refers to not being able to interpret sensations and hence to recognize things. Recognition impairments can be evident if there are concerns during the examination about the patient's ability to recognize stimuli using their senses of vision, hearing, tactile function, or olfaction. Agnosia is relatively common in Alzheimer's disease, frontotemporal dementia, Lewy body dementia, and Parkinson's disease with dementia. The most common type of agnosia is visual.

Since an agnosia must be distinguished from anomia, a detailed language examination during the mental status examination is required. If consultation is needed, a speech-language specialist or occupational therapist experienced in these matters may be useful (Holzer et al., 2018).

Common agnosias

- **Object agnosia** - inability to recognize objects
- **Form agnosia** - inability to recognize a whole object due to failure to recognize one of its parts
- **Shape agnosia** - inability to recognize the shape of an object despite ability to recognize its color, size, etc.
- **Finger agnosia** - inability to recognize fingers on the hands (a component of German syndrome: agraphia, acalculia, left-right disorientation, finger agnosia)
- **Mirror agnosia** - inability to recognize objects or activity in the right or left field of view
- **Pure word blindness** - inability to read despite preserved perception of words and sentences (the person can copy text that he/she "can't read")
- **Color agnosia** - inability to recognize colors despite the ability to distinguish red from green, blue from yellow, etc.
- **Simultanagnosia** - inability to synthesize multiple visual elements despite recognizing individual elements (e.g. of a painting)
- **Prosopagnosia** - inability to recognize previously familiar faces
- **Auditory agnosia** - inability to recognize environmental sounds, such as a barking dog or an automobile engine
- **Tactile agnosia** - inability to recognize objects by touch or writing onto the hand or fingertips
- **Anosognosia** - inability to recognize disease in one's self

Holzer et al., 2018

Aphasia

Aphasia refers to loss of ability to understand or express speech, involving impairments in one or more of the four principle components of language: fluency, repetition, comprehension, and/or naming. Imagine a geriatric forensic examinee with a substantial aphasia, who cannot comprehend oral or written language, being asked to engage in a contractual matter, consent to surgery, or produce a valid will. Proper use of language is essential for any issue of competency before a forensic psychiatrist, and assessment of language often includes an evaluation of ability to comprehend, repeat, name, follow commands, speak with fluency, and provide prosody (the rhythm, stress, and intonation of speech, produced in parallel with the narrative as one of the affective components of speech.)

Components of language that can be impaired in aphasia

- Fluency
- Repetition
- Naming

In an older person, aphasic disorders can have multiple etiologies, including traumatic brain injury (TBI), stroke, brain tumor, infection, and dementias.

Degenerative types of aphasia

Progressive aphasias

- Degenerative forms of aphasia, such as seen in the dementias, are referred to as progressive aphasias, as they progress with the disease process. For example, primary progressive aphasia often accompanies frontotemporal dementia. Broce's aphasia (also termed expressive or motor aphasia), is usually found in those diseases producing lesions in or near the left medial insular cortex. In contrast, damage usually found in the left temporal lobe may result in a fluent Wernicke's aphasia (also termed sensory or receptive aphasia)

Other forms of aphasia

- Pure word deafness
- Conduction aphasia
- Global aphasia
- Transcortical aphasias
- Anomic aphasia - common in Alzheimer's diseases

Source: Holzer et al., 2018

The forensic psychiatrist should consider enlisting the aid of a neuropsychologist or speech and language pathologist if language evaluation is required within the psychiatrist's forensic assessment of an elderly person. The Boston Diagnostic Aphasia Examination (BDAE) is an example of a test for measuring deficits of language.

If the forensic psychiatrist is using the Mini Mental State Examination (MMSE) as part of the assessment process, it should be noted that the three-step comprehension task on the MMSE is actually a test of ideational praxis, and impaired performance on it requires dissection of the patient's performance into its language- and praxis-related components.

Apraxia

Apraxia refers to inability to perform particular purposive action, denotes impairment of this ability that cannot be attributed to any sensory, motor, or language disturbances (praxis refers to the ability to perform skilled, purposeful movements on demand). It is a relatively common feature of various neurodegenerative disorders. Apraxia may involve various parts of the motor system, including axial, limb, and/or whole-body movements.

Types of praxis that may a concern in an older individual

The major types of apraxia

- **Limb kinetic**: inability to execute precise individual finger movements on demand (not universally accepted as a true apraxia)
- **Ideomotor**: inability to pantomime movements to verbal command despite preservation of the same movements in a naturalistic setting
- **Ideational**: inability to carry out a complex series of movements despite the ability to perform individual components (e.g. "fold a piece of paper; carry it across the room; place it on the coffee table")

Adapted from Holzer et al., 2018; Squire, 1987

Ideomotor apraxia frequently involves both axial and limb movements. Ideational apraxia occurs most often in a setting of acute confusional states seen in the dementias and other disorders that affect frontal-subcortical function. It overlaps clinically with impairments of executive function and/or attention.

Geriatric forensic issues related to apraxia

- Apraxia may adversely affect the examinee's ability to make use of his/her other cognitive functions (whether they are intact or impaired)
- Apraxia may diminish functional status

DSM-5 neurocognitive disorders

In 2013, the APA published the fifth Edition of the Diagnostic and Statistical Manual of Mental Disorders (DSM-5). Dementia has been renamed 'major neurocognitive disorder' in the DSM-5 and it recognizes earlier stages of cognitive decline as 'mild neurocognitive disorder'. The aims of this reclassification included:

- reducing stigma associated with the term "dementia", especially for younger people
- bringing the diagnostic guidelines into line with current clinical practice

The intention was to not to eliminate the term dementia entirely from the nomenclature but to subsume entities currently known as dementia under the broad category of major NCDs (American Psychiatric and American Psychiatric Association, 2013). Some have suggested to include the term dementia in parentheses. In this way, it can continue to be used in groups where dementia is the standard term, as in AD, without being imposed in settings where it is not customary (Sachdev et al., 2014). The major NCD term is broader than dementia however (American Psychiatric Association, 2013).

A clear understanding of the spectrum of DSM-5 Neurocognitive disorders and of their diagnosis is imperative for geriatric forensic evaluators. DSM-5 conceptualizes mild neurocognitive disorder as a new entity. The previously common diagnosis of cognitive disorder, not otherwise specified is eliminated in DSM-5. Algorithms at end of this chapter will summarize how to apply the diagnostic labels. Readers are also encouraged to refer to the full DSM-5 manual for additional details.

General diagnostic criteria

Neurocognitive disorders (NCD)

- Primarily COGNITIVE disorders
- Acquired and represent decline (i.e. not developmental)
- Underlying brain pathology
- For degenerative disorders monitor consensus guidelines in addition to DSM 5

Cognitive domains

Whereas DSM-IV-TR (2000) focused on memory impairment along with aphasia, apraxia, agnosia, and executive dysfunction, DSM-5 (2013) introduced 6 new cognitive domains of DSM-5. Only one is required for Major NCD, except for Alzheimer's disease which requires 2 domains.

Cognitive domains in mild and major NCD

- **Complex attention** - sustained attention, divided attention, selective attention, and information processing speed
- **Executive function** - planning, decision making, working memory, responding to feedback, inhibition, mental flexibility
- **Learning and memory** - free recall, cued recall, recognition memory, semantic and autobiographical long-term memory, implicit learning
- **Language** - object naming, word finding, fluency, grammar and syntax, receptive language
- **Perceptual-motor function** - visual perception, visuo-constructional reasoning, perceptual-motor coordination
- **Social cognition** - recognition of emotions, theory of mind, insight

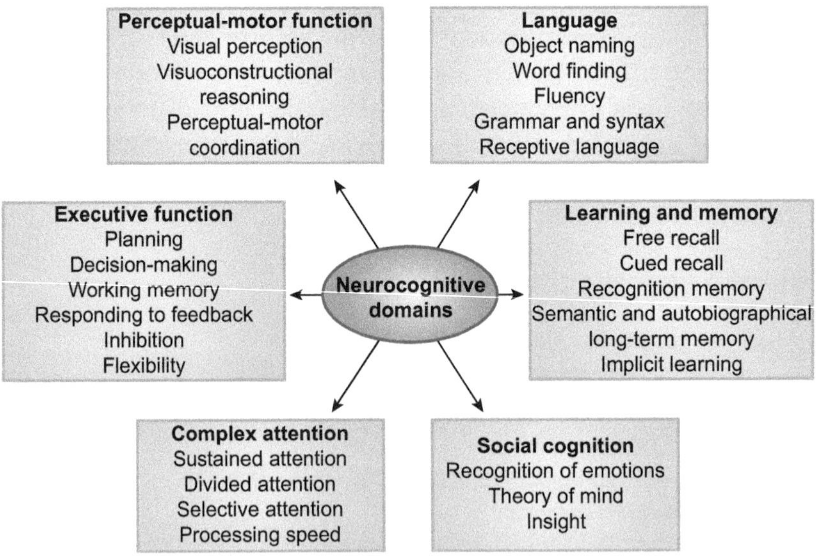

From American Psychiatric, A. and D. S. M. T. F. American Psychiatric Association (2013). Diagnostic and statistical manual of mental disorders: DSM-5. Arlington, Va., Arlington, Va.: American Psychiatric Association. Reprinted with permission from the Diagnostic and Statistical Manual of Mental Disorders, Fifth Edition, (Copyright ©2013). American Psychiatric Association. All Rights Reserved.

Clinicians evaluating for dementia may note symptoms of the 6 domains in many ways. Deficits in the 6 domains can show up with a wide variety of presentations.

To point out a few examples, an individual with major or mild neurocognitive disorder may have deficits in complex attention (e.g. increased difficulty in environments with multiple stimuli), executive function (needs to rely on others to plan activities of daily living or make decisions), learning and memory (repeats self, difficulty recalling recent events), language (uses general-use phrases such as "that thing" and "you know what I mean," prefers general pronouns rather than names), perceptual-motor (difficulties with previously familiar activities like using tools, driving), social cognition (changes in behavior or attitude, often described as a change in personality, or behavior clearly out of acceptable social range; insensitivity to social standards and typically poor insight into these changes).

More details and examples of questions a clinician might ask to evaluate the 6 neurocognitive domains are included in the main text of DSM-5 (American Psychiatric Association, 2013).

Psychometric definitions

For major NCD, performance is typically 2 or more standard deviations below appropriate norms, and for mild NCD, performance typically lies in the 1–2 standard deviation range. These categories should not be rigidly used, since in clinical populations major and mild NCD exist on a continuum. In interpreting test results, clinicians should consider the patient's premorbid functioning level, education, and sensitivity of the tests being used.

Neuropsychological testing is not formally required to diagnose NCD according to DSM-5. However, it can be a part of a standard evaluation of NCDs. Norms should be carefully chosen to be appropriate to the patient's age, educational attainment, and background. It can be more challenging to interpret in individuals with very high or very low levels of education or with a different language or culture.

Neuropsychological testing can be particularly helpful in cases of suspected mild NCD, where deficits are often subtle. Where neuropsychological testing is unavailable or infeasible, a variety of brief office-based or "bedside" assessments such as the Montreal Cognitive Assessment (MOCA), Mini Mental State Examination (MMSE) or the Mini-Cog can also supply objective data. Such tests are discussed in more detail later in this chapter.

Psychometric definitions for mild versus major NCD

- Mild: 1–2 standard deviation (SD) range (between the third and 16th percentiles)
- Major: Below 2 SD or third percentile

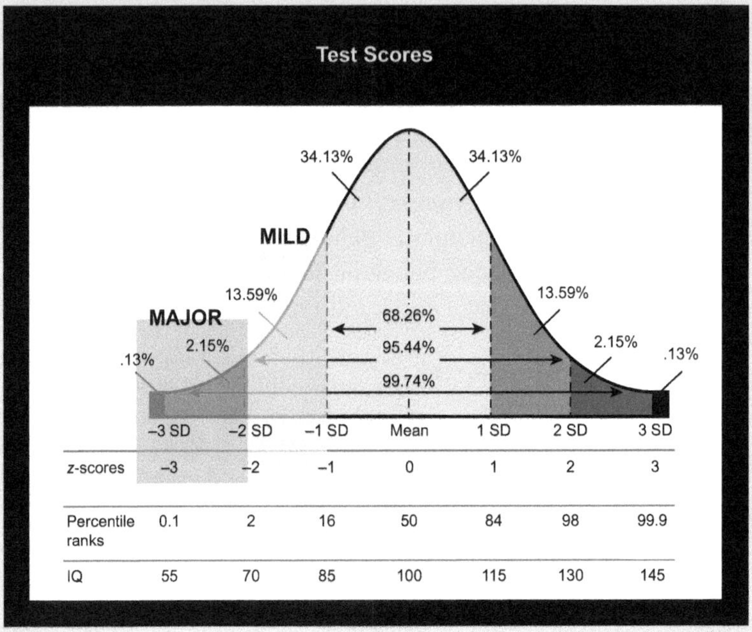

Rosen (2017).

Etiological subtypes of NCDs

Major and mild neurocognitive disorders (NCDs) are primarily subtyped according to the known or presumed etiological/pathological entity or entities underlying the cognitive decline. These subtypes are distinguished on the basis of a combination of time course, characteristic domains affected, and associated symptoms.

For certain etiological subtypes, the diagnosis depends substantially on the presence of a potentially causative entity, such as Parkinson's or Huntington's disease, or a traumatic brain injury or stroke in the appropriate time period. For other etiological subtypes (generally the neurodegenerative diseases like Alzheimer's disease, frontotemporal lobar degeneration, and Lewy body disease), the diagnosis is based primarily on the cognitive, behavioral, and functional symptoms.

Typically, the differentiation among these syndromes that lack an independently recognized etiological entity is clearer at the level of major NCD than at the level of mild NCD, but sometimes characteristic symptoms and associated features are present at the mild level as well.

Diagnosing mild or major NCD should be followed by an examination of potential causes so that a subtype can be assigned. In many people with NCDs, there is evidence of a causative disorder, such as Huntington's disease or HIV infection. In others, the cognitive symptoms emerge first and progression provides evidence of a causative disorder such as Alzheimer's disease or Lewy body disease. In many cases, especially with older people, there are multiple causative factors, and the diagnosis should recognize this. Subtypes of minor and major NCD in the DSM-5 include:

DSM-5 NCD subtypes

- Major or Mild Neurocognitive Disorder Due to **Alzheimer's Disease**
- Major or Mild **Frontotemporal** Neurocognitive Disorder
- Major or Mild Neurocognitive Disorder with **Lewy Bodies**
- Major or Mild **Vascular** Neurocognitive Disorder
- Major or Mild Neurocognitive Disorder Due to **Traumatic Brain Injury**
- **Substance/Medication-Induced** Major or Mild Neurocognitive Disorder
- Major or Mild Neurocognitive Disorder Due to **HIV Infection**
- Major or Mild Neurocognitive Disorder Due to **Prion Disease**
- Major or Mild Neurocognitive Disorder Due to **Parkinson's Disease**
- Major or Mild Neurocognitive Disorder Due to **Huntington's Disease**
- Major or Mild Neurocognitive Disorder Due to **Another Medical Condition**
- Major or Mild Neurocognitive Disorder Due to **Multiple Etiologies**
- **Unspecified** Neurocognitive Disorder

(DSM-5, American Psychiatric Association, 2013)

Creutzfeldt-Jacob disease is remarkable in that it usually presents as a rapidly progressive dementia with aphasia, amnesia, apraxia, and agnosia. The average forensic psychiatrist will never see a case of this, as it has a worldwide incidence of approximately one per million. Ninety percent of cases arise sporadically.

Unspecified neurocognitive disorder

Applies to presentations in which symptoms characteristic of a neurocognitive disorder that cause clinically significant distress or impairment in social, occupational, or other important areas of functioning predominate but do not meet the full criteria for any of the disorders in the neurocognitive disorders diagnostic

(Continued)

Unspecified neurocognitive disorder (*cont'd*)

class. Used in situations in which the precise etiology cannot be determined with sufficient certainty to make an etiological attribution (American Psychiatric Association, 2013).

Major and mild neurocognitive disorders

Major neurocognitive disorder

Diagnosis of major NCD requires evidence of significant cognitive decline from a previous level of performance in one or more of the cognitive domains outlined above. Additionally, the cognitive deficits must be sufficient to interfere with independence in activities of daily living. The cognitive deficits must not be attributable to another mental disorder. The criterion of maintenance or loss of independent functioning represents the key distinction between mild and major NCD. Algorithm at end of chapter will demonstrate how to apply diagnostic labels. Refer to DSM-5 for additional details.

Major NCD criteria

- Significant Cognitive Decline
- Interferes with independence
- Not due to delirium
- Not due to other mental disorder

Major NCD versus Dementia

Can be single domain

- e.g. Amnestic
- Exception: Major NCD due to Alzheimer's disease requires 2 domains

---

Memory impairment no longer a requirement for Major NCD, except in cases of Alzheimer's disease where 2 domains are still required, one of which must be memory impairment.

Diagnosis of dementia (NCD) can be made without overt memory impairments, except in cases of Alzheimer's where two domains are still required, one of which must be memory impairment. Impairment in only one cognitive domain is enough to qualify for a diagnosis of a major NCD.

There is a growing recognition that a significant percentage of people with NCDs, particularly frontotemporal dementia, have a relatively intact memory, at least until later in the course of illness, which is likely to be important in both civil and criminal forensic criminal forensic matters (Simpson, 2014).

Major and mild NCD descriptors

- Possible versus probable
- Behavioral Disturbance
  a) With: e.g. psychosis, mood, agitation
  b) Without (not clinically significant Older subjects actually perform better on some memory tests, an effect that may be attributed to increased overall knowledge
- Severity (level of disability)
  a) Mild: Instrumental ADL's are preserved
  b) Moderate: Basic ADL's affected– Severe: Fully dependent

Basic and instrumental activities of daily living (ADLs)

- Basic ADLs: self-care tasks usually learned in childhood such as walking, feeding, dressing and grooming, toileting, transferring
- Instrumental ADLs (IADLs): self care tasks usually learned as a teenager such as managing finances, transportation, shopping and meal preparation, housecleaning and home maintenance

Mild neurocognitive disorder

Mild NCD is a new diagnostic category in the DSM-5, added to recognize the substantial clinical needs of individuals living with this disorder, which might also be termed Mild Cognitive Impairment (MCI) or prodromal dementia. Diagnosis of MCI has become increasingly common in clinical practice, partly because people with cognitive decline are seeking assessment and treatment earlier, before a diagnosis of dementia is justified.

The move to diagnose NCDs as early as possible also emerged from the recognition of a long pre-dementia stage in neurodegenerative diseases such as Alzheimer's, improvements in early diagnosis, and the increasing emphasis on early intervention to prevent or postpone dementia. Importantly, mild

NCD is not always a precursor of major NCD, and the diagnosis does not require further decline. There may be continued decline, as in neurodegenerative diseases, or the impairment may be static or even improve, as in traumatic brain injury.

Diagnosis of mild NCD requires evidence of modest cognitive decline from a previous level of performance in one or more of the cognitive domains outlined above. These cognitive deficits must be insufficient to interfere with independence in daily activities, although greater effort and compensatory strategies may be required to maintain the level of independence. Further, the cognitive deficits must not be due to another mental disorder (such as depression).

Mild NCD

- Like Mild Cognitive Impairment (MCI)
- Previously: Cognitive Disorder Not Otherwise Specified
- Cognitive impairments that are not severe enough to qualify for a diagnosis of dementia
- Continuum between mild and major NCDs, differ in degree, not in kind
- TBI, stroke, anoxia, acute toxic exposure
- Mild NCDs sounds more definitive, may carry more weight in courtroom, more difficult to discount in a legal context
- What is the impact of mild NCD on other functional or legal capabilities? Can mild NCD render someone incompetent or incapacitated?
- Actual effect of these changes on fact finders is not known

Simpson 2014

Mild NCD criteria

- Moderate Cognitive Decline
- Does NOT interfere with independence
- Not due to delirium
- Not due to other mental disorder

With regards to the practice of forensic psychiatry, one potential change introduced with the new NCD categorization in DSM-5 is that the severe, disabling cognitive disorders (the dementias) may more clearly be viewed as lying on a continuum with the less severe disorders that do not reach the threshold for a diagnosis of dementia. The new classification system may prove useful in emphasizing that mild NCDs differ from major NCDs only in degree, not in kind. In many cases, mild NCD will unfortunately be nothing more than a transitional state on the inexorable path to a major NCD (Simpson, 2014).

For NCD due to TBI specified in DSM-5, and for post-concussional syndromes such as chronic traumatic encephalopathy (CTE), a diagnosis of mild NCD sounds more definitive and therefore may carry more weight in the courtroom than the former cognitive disorder NOS.

The recognition that some patients with dementia have relatively intact memory is also likely to be important in both civil and criminal forensic matters.

Patients whose dementia manifests in impaired judgment and executive function, but whose memory is intact, may now be identified more easily, and the impact of their impaired condition on their legal capacities may be better appreciated (Simpson, 2014).

Delirium

Delirium is a physiological consequence of medical conditions, substance intake, withdrawal from medication, and toxicity from medication. It has a rapid onset from hours to days. Symptoms can include confusion, hallucinations, and agitation. An older person with delirium will often seem bewildered and disoriented, asking, where am I?

Delirium diagnostic criteria

- Rapid and abrupt onset of:
  a) Impaired Attention
  b) Lack of Awareness of environment
- Change in at least ONE Cognitive Domain:
  a) Recent Memory
  b) Orientation
  c) Language (i.e. rambled speech, mumbling, difficult to understand)
  d) Perceptual Disturbance
- Associated features:
  a) Change in sleep-wake cycle
  b) Change in emotional states– Worsening of behavioral problems in the evening

How delirium differs from other NCDs

- Rapid onset: hours to days
- Linked to medical condition, substance intoxication/withdrawal, medications, other causes
- May resolve completely
- Symptom length
  a) Acute-hours to days
  b) Persistent-weeks to months

DSM-5 Attenuated delirium syndrome

- Example of the diagnosis other specified delirium
- Severity of cognitive impairment falls short of that required for the diagnosis (i.e. only some of the criteria for delirium are met)

The lucid interval

The "lucid interval" is a legal concept that refers to a brief period during which an insane person regains sanity that is sufficient to regain the legal capacity to contract and to act on his/her own behalf.

The lucid interval is a long-held legal concept widely accepted in case law as a possible means of countering a challenge to testamentary and related capacities. In parallel, the clinical phenomenon of cognitive fluctuations has been considered a common element of several neurodegenerative disorders (dementias), including Alzheimer Disease, but is especially prevalent in vascular dementia and dementia with Lewy bodies.

Shulman et al. 2015

Cognitive fluctuations in dementia largely affect attention and alertness, rather than memory or the higher-level executive functions.

Interview tips for Delirium (Gibson, 2017).

- Always tell the person who you are and why you are there.
- Person will not be able to make sense of your presence.
- Person wiIl not be able to repeat what you told them
- Person will appear bewildered, " Where am I, what are you doing here?"
- Person will be difficult to console

- His/her conversation will likely contain suspiciousness; seem panicky, emotional, or pressured
- Person will be difficult to "connect" with during the interview
- Person will tend to misinterpret what he or she sees and hears (e.g. thread on the couch is a snake)

Conversational Clues to Delirium in a forensic interview (cite Gibson).

- Unable to answer "Where are we right now?" or "What day/time/date is it?"
- Can they engage in meaningful dialogue?
- Do they appear aware of their surroundings? Are they able to focus?

Tips for diagnosing dementia and DSM-5 NCDs

Interviewing strategies

For interviews in dementia, depending on the stage of dementia, the person will likely be able to understand and give a basic explanation of why you were there.

In early to middle stages, you may notice vague speech and other symptoms as noted in the text box.

Features of early to middle stage dementia and a clinical interview

- Vague speech, when asked why you are (?) that a person might say "there must be a problem"
- Repeated phrases
- Losing track during conversation, uses storytelling instead of logical presentation of facts, devolves into narrative of storytelling
- May not be troubled by mistakes or will lack awareness of incorrect answers
- May make excuses for why he or she cannot perform a task or answer a question
- May present as excessively friendly or hostile

Gibson 2017

Differential diagnosis of dementias

Dementia is a general term for loss of memory and other mental abilities severe enough to interfere with daily life, caused by physical changes in the brain. There are many different kinds of dementia. A mixed etiology is likely the most common cause of dementia. Though Alzheimer's disease is the most common form of dementia, all dementia is not Alzheimer's disease.

Alzheimer's disease is the most common form of dementia, but all dementia is not Alzheimer's disease.

Differential diagnosis of major dementias

Disease	First symptoms	Early cognitive changes	Neuropsychiatric symptoms
Alzheimer's disease	Memory loss	Episodic memory loss	Initially normal, later apathy, disinhibition
Frontotemporal Dementia (FTD)	Apathy; poor judgment/ insight, speech problems; hyperorality	Frontal/ executive, language	Apathy, disinhibition, hyperorality, euphoria, depression
Dementia with Lewy Bodies (DLB)	Visual hallucinations, REM sleep disorder, delirium, Capgras syndrome, parkinsonism	Visuospatial, frontal/ executive; memory is relatively spared; delirium risk	Visual hallucinations, depression, sleep disorder, delusions
Creutzfeldt-Jakob disease (CJD)	Dementia, mood, anxiety, movement disorders	Memory, frontal/ executive	Depression, anxiety
Vascular Dementia	Often but not always sudden; variable; apathy, falls, focal weakness	Frontal/ executive, cognitive slowing; can spare memory	Apathy, delusions, anxiety

Dementia is a clinical diagnosis

Dementia is primarily a clinical diagnosis, based on the clinician's overall judgment, integrating many factors. No single test, including cognitive screening tests such as the popular Mini Mental State Examination (MMSE), can on its own reliably diagnose Alzheimer's and rule out differential diagnostic considerations. Clinicians diagnosing dementia must consider myriad factors including the longitudinal history, medical status, medications, physical and mental status examination, and much more.

> *Dementia is primarily a clinical diagnosis, based on the clinician's overall judgment, integrating many factors.*

For many practicing forensic psychiatrists and psychologists, diagnosing dementia, determining its severity, and reaching a conclusion about its effect on the medicolegal capacity in question is a regular component of their work. As the average age of the population continues to increase in most industrialized countries, the demand for mental health professionals who have the expertise in dementia to address medicolegal concerns is certain to grow (Simpson, 2014).

As explored further, later in this chapter, the revised diagnostic nomenclature for the Diagnostic and Statistical Manual of Mental Disorders, Fifth Edition, or DSM-5 (American Psychiatric Association, 2013) replaces the term dementia with Major or Minor Neurocognitive Disorder (NCD) to provide a broader definition.

Classification of Alzheimer's disease in DSM-5

Dementia caused by AD can be further classified as:

- Probable Alzheimer's disease dementia, to be diagnosed when the person meets all the core clinical criteria
- Possible Alzheimer's disease dementia, to be diagnosed when there is an atypical or mixed presentation
- Probable or possible Alzheimer's disease dementia, with evidence of the Alzheimer's disease pathological process, to be diagnosed when there is biomarker evidence to increase the certainty that the dementia is due to Alzheimer's disease

Diagnostic tests for dementia and role of neuroimaging/biomarkers

Elements of a diagnostic workup for Dementia

- Clinical examination (most types of dementia can be diagnosed based on consensus criteria)
- Medical history
- Mental status examination
- Cognitive testing with assessment of multiple cognitive domains
- Lab tests
- MRI and/or CT scan, in some cases

Biomarkers may be increasingly used to help improve diagnostic certainty, especially for research purposes. Biomarkers, both chemical and imaging, are indicators of specific changes that characterize AD in vivo. Evidence suggests that these AD biomarkers do not reach abnormal levels or peak simultaneously but do so in an ordered manner. Measurement of these biomarkers in longitudinal observational studies is now commonplace, enabling investigators to establish the correct ordering of the relevant biomarkers and their relationships to clinical symptoms (Jack et al., 2010).

In distinguishing among etiological subtypes, additional diagnostic markers may come into play, particularly neuroimaging studies such as magnetic resonance imaging scans and positron emission tomography scans. In addition, specific markers may be involved in the assessment of specific subtypes and may become more important as additional research findings accumulate over time, as discussed in the relevant sections.

Text Box: Alzheimer's Pathological Cascade (Figs. 3.1 and 3.2).

Three elderly individuals are placed in order from left to right by use of our proposed biomarker staging scheme. (A) A cognitively normal individual with no evidence of Aβ on PET amyloid imaging with PiB and no evidence of atrophy on MRI. (B) A cognitively normal individual who has no evidence of neurodegenerative atrophy on MRI, but has significant Aβ deposition on PET amyloid imaging. (B) An individual who has dementia and a clinical diagnosis of Alzheimer's disease, a positive PET amyloid imaging study, and neurodegenerative atrophy on MRI. Aβ = β-amyloid. PiB = Pittsburgh compound B (Jack et al., 2010).

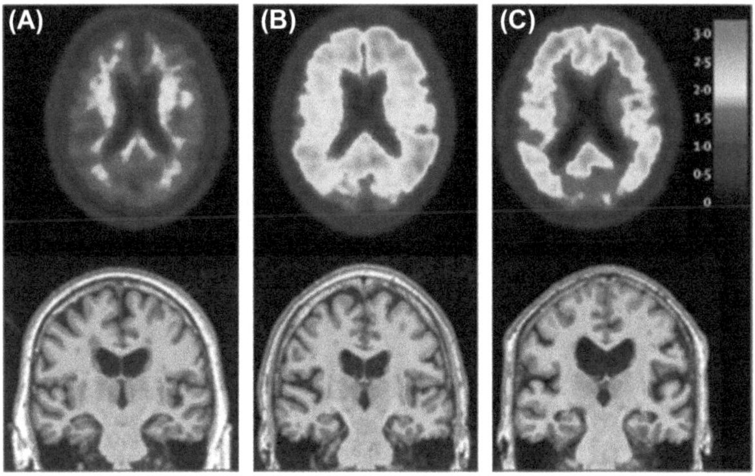

Fig. 3.1 Dynamic biomarkers of the Alzheimer's pathological cascade. *From Jack, C. R., D. S. Knopman, W. J. Jagust, L. M. Shaw, P. S. Aisen, M. W. Weiner, R. C. Petersen and J. Q. Trojanowski (2010). "Hypothetical model of dynamic biomarkers of the Alzheimer's pathological cascade." Lancet Neurology 9(1): 119–128. Reprinted with permission from Elsevier (The Lancet, 2010, 9, 119–128).*

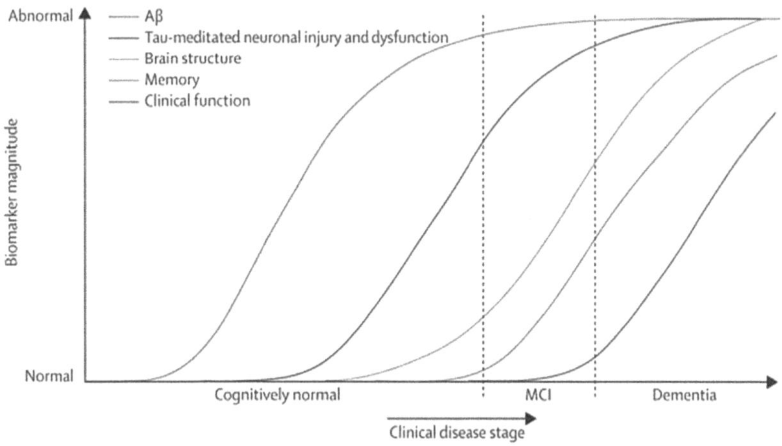

Fig. 3.2 Illustration of biomarker staging of Alzheimer's disease. *From Jack, C. R., D. S. Knopman, W. J. Jagust, L. M. Shaw, P. S. Aisen, M. W. Weiner, R. C. Petersen and J. Q. Trojanowski (2010). "Hypothetical model of dynamic biomarkers of the Alzheimer's pathological cascade." Lancet Neurology 9(1): 119–128. Reprinted with permission from Elsevier (The Lancet, 2010, 9, 119–128).*

Without necessarily resulting from pathological findings, advanced neuroimaging can produce distracting colorful images that dazzle — and distract - the viewer, a tendency sometimes referred to as the "Christmas tree effect."

Aβ is identified by CSF $A\beta_{42}$ or PET amyloid imaging. Tau-mediated neuronal injury and dysfunction is identified by CSF tau or fluorodeoxyglucose-PET. Brain structure is measured by use of structural MRI. Aβ = β-amyloid. MCI = mild cognitive impairment (Jack, 2010).

The gold standard for diagnosis of dementia is autopsy - pathological examination of the brain.

The gold standard for diagnosis of dementia is autopsy, pathological examination of the brain, but non-invasive imaging techniques such as CT or MRI may provide useful information about the functional integrity of brain. Currently, imaging techniques are not sufficient to diagnose dementia, though they may provide information in a clinical context. Data from brain scans is challenging to interpret, and for individual cases the information obtained from imaging is rarely helpful to inform the diagnostic question or treatment decision. Many individuals with abnormal scans are cognitively intact, and many with normal scans have cognitive deficits. This is an active area of research.

Diagnosing DSM-5 neurocognitive disorders

Note unwieldy use of adjective "mild"

The mild-major continuum will undoubtedly take some getting used to. Under the new schema, any cause of dementia can also produce mild NCD. Thus, both major and mild NCD due to Alzheimer's disease are diagnosable conditions. Clinicians may find it awkward to apply the Alzheimer's label to patients who do not meet criteria for dementia, as Alzheimer's has heretofore been essentially synonymous with senile dementia.

This type of usage may be less confusing for mild NCD due to, for example, Parkinson's or Huntington's disease, in which other symptoms are often much more prominent than the cognitive impairments, particularly early in the course of illness. Potentially adding to the confusion, the term mild has been retained as a specifier of severity for the major NCDs, along with moderate and severe (Simpson, 2014).

For example, in DSM-5 we find this sentence: "Apathy is common in mild and mild major NCD." It seems unwieldy that the same adjective, mild, can be used either in reference to an NCD not severe enough to qualify as a dementia or when describing the severity of a particular clinical case of dementia (i.e. a major NCD). In other words, a patient can have mild NCD (not a dementia), mild major NCD, moderate major NCD, or severe major NCD (these latter three are all dementias). In theory, a patient might even progress through each of these stages over time. Granted, the mild major usage is not much different from the use of the mild specifier in major depressive disorder, but it seems to risk confusion among providers as well as consumers and their family members nonetheless.

A further potential source of confusion or ambiguity of the NCD conceptualization is that for several of the most common dementia syndromes, the clinician is expected to qualify the diagnosis with the descriptor probable or possible. This is the case for those NCDs that lack a gold standard premortem diagnostic test, specifically: Alzheimer's disease, frontotemporal lobar degeneration (Pick's disease in DSM-IV and DSM-IV-TR), Lewy Body disease, vascular disease, and Parkinson's disease. In cases of NCD due to traumatic brain injury (TBI), HIV infection, prion disease, or Huntington's disease, the probable and possible specifiers are not required, as the causative (Simpson, 2014).

"Mild major" usage risks confusion

The mild major usage seems to risk confusion, since the same adjective, mild, is used either in reference to:

- NCD not severe enough to qualify as a dementia, **mild NCD**
- Describing the severity of a particular clinical case of dementia, i.e. a major NCD, **mild major NCD**

In other words, a patient can have:

- **Mild NCD (not a dementia)**
- **Mild major NCD**
- **Moderate major NCD**
- **Severe major NCD** (latter three are all dementia)

In theory, the same patient might progress through all of these stages over time.

Simpson 2014

Algorithms for DSM-5 NCD diagnosis

Check DSM-5 for precise wording of each etiological subtype	Probable	Possible
Major NCD	Probable Major Neurocognitive Disorder due to ______	Possible Major Neurocognitive Disorder due to ______
Mild NCD	Probable Mild Neurocognitive Disorder due to ______	Possible Mild Neurocognitive Disorder due to ______

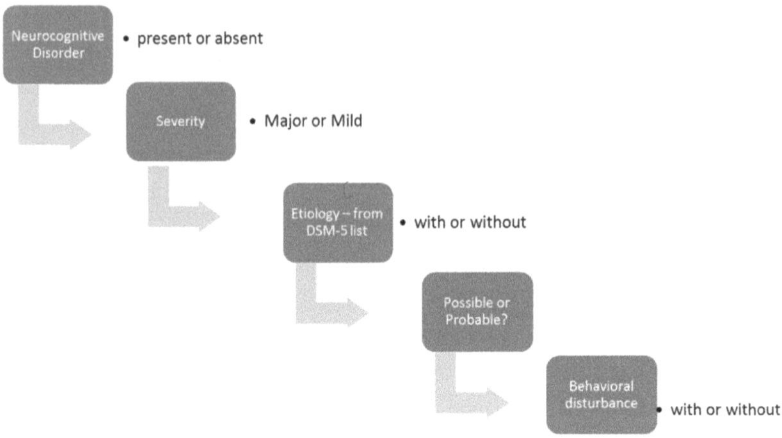

Cognitive screening in older adults

Screening tools for cognition, such as the Mini Mental State Examination and MSC, the Montréal Cognitive Assessment (MoCA), and the Executive Interview (EXIT) are available. In some cases, formal neuropsychological testing, involving quantitative evaluation of various cognitive spheres of functioning, may be indicated as part of a workup for MCI or dementia. The gold standard for assessment of executive function is traditional neuropsychological testing, which offers the most detailed picture of an individual's cognition.

Unfortunately, formal neuropsychological testing is time-consuming and requires specially trained personnel, advanced test material, and a structured setting. It is typically performed over an extended appointment lasting several hours, using comprehensive batteries and specialized tests for specific aspects of executive function such as response inhibition (Stroop Color/Word Interference Test), set shifting (Wisconsin Card Sorting Test), divided attention (Trail Making Part B), and productivity and flexibility (fluency tests).

The gold standard for assessment of cognitive domains is traditional neuropsychological testing.

Selecting a cognitive screening test

Cognitive screening instruments may be encountered by practitioners in many branches of clinical medicine, in both primary and secondary care. However, not all clinicians may feel themselves either familiar with or competent in the use of such instruments. This may stem in part from lack of appropriate training, and exacerbated by the profusion of potential tests available.

The "best" cognitive screening instrument depends on multiple factors including the clinical circumstances and the evaluation setting.

Shorter screening tools can provide easier, reliable, and quicker measures of executive function that can be useful in initial or follow up clinical assessments, where time and resources are limited. A physician or other team member (e.g. therapist, nurse, social worker) can use an executive function screening tool for initial executive function evaluation. If a problem in cognition is identified during the screening, additional physician evaluation and formal neuropsychological assessment can be arranged.

Despite its prevalent use, especially for people with dementia, the Mini Mental Status Exam (MMSE) does not assess executive function impairment, requiring other tools to detect this important and complex range of cognitive, emotional and behavioral difficulties.

The popular Mini Mental Status Exam (MMSE) does ***not*** *assess executive function.*

In clinical practice, executive function screening tests can help clinicians identify cognitive impairment early, which is important since cognitive impairment often progresses to dementia eventually. Screening instruments can be used to establish a baseline, guide decisions regarding the need for further cognitive assessment, and monitor treatment.

While standardized screening instruments such as the MMSE, MoCA and Clock Drawing Test (CDT) are of clinical value, they must be viewed and interpreted with caution in the context of a capacity assessment.

Early identification of executive function deficits can help clinicians optimize the patient's future function, safety, and emotional well-being. It can allow for planning of future changes to the patient's living environment and caregiver support, including completing advance directives and establishing medical and financial proxy decision makers.

Screening tests that ***do*** *include assessment of executive function in older people include the Montreal Cognitive Assessment (MOCA), St. Louis University Mental Status Examination (SLUMS), Clock Drawing Test (CDT), Frontal Assessment Battery (FAB), and Executive Interview (EXIT).*

Selected instruments

A good cognitive screening test should assess several cognitive domains in order to cast as wide a net as possible and hopefully not miss a specific area of impairment. Fortunately, there are other clinical tools in the public domain offering improved screening for executive function deficits, compared with the MMSE. The following executive function tests are widely available and can be quickly administered by a variety of disciplines.

Assessment in dementia relies on collateral as well as patient-derived information. Many assessment scales have been developed over decades for use in dementia research and care. These scales are used to reduce uncertainty in decision making, for example in screening for cognitive impairment, making diagnoses of dementia, and monitoring change. Ideal scales used in dementia should demonstrate face validity and concurrent validity against gold standard assessments, should be reliable, practical, and should rely on objective rather than subjective information.

This section will review selected screening tools for cognition that are currently available and can be important in assessing an elderly evaluee for cognitive deficits. If the above initial screening tests suggest deficits, it may be helpful to employ more specialized tests specifically developed to assess executive function.

Calculation, verbal fluency, naming

Calculation, verbal fluency, and naming are routinely used to evaluate cognitive function in older adults. Verbal fluency tests assess spontaneous ability to generate words under certain circumstances and within time constraints.

Clock drawing test (CDT)

Clock drawing has become one of the standard cognitive screening tools used around the world. It is easy to administer, displays good inter-rater reliability, is strongly associated with cognitive test scores, requires minimal equipment, is portable, quick and can be administered to the hearing impaired, the very ill and the poorly educated. The CDT (Clock-Drawing Test) or CLOX (Executive Clock-Drawing Task) (Royall, 1998) takes only 2–3 min to administer and assesses cognitive or visuospatial impairment. The patient is simply asked to draw the face of a clock, including the numbers, and then to place the hands to designate a certain time, such as "10 min after eleven." Scoring is based on features such as size, spacing and placement of numbers or hands, disorganization, perseveration, completeness, and other errors indicating cognitive impairment. (Mainland and Shulman, 2013).

Instruct the older person to set the time to "10 past 11". Individuals with cognitive impairment often 'pull' the minute hand to point to '10' rather than '2'.

Drawing a clock requires multiple cognitive functions (not just visuospatial ability). It requires: visual memory of a clock; planning ability and concentration in order to place the numbers evenly around the clock circle; and abstract ability to set the time using the symbol of hands which point to the number 2 to represent 10 min past the hour. The latter task is very sensitive to cognitive impairment as affected individuals often 'pull' the minute hand to point to the number 10 rather than 2.

Clock-drawing correlates very well with the MMSE. It takes less time to administer and is generally very well accepted. It is as sensitive to cognitive impairment as the MMSE and picks up changes in cognition over time. Moreover, it tests frontal-executive higher-level brain functioning (abstract ability) in a way that the MMSE does not. Also, the visual impact of abnormal clocks is often an eye opener for families who may not have been aware of the full extent of cognitive dysfunction. The clock test is frequently used in combination with the MMSE as a screening battery (Shulman, 2018).

Clock drawing is of course subject to the same limitations as all screening tests, including the MMSE. It is affected by level of education and should not be used alone for diagnostic purposes or for assessing the severity of cognitive impairment. However, like all good screening tests it does tap into multiple cognitive functions and can provide a 'signal' that calls for further inquiry or more investigations. Importantly, it also establishes a baseline for future monitoring to determine if cognitive impairment is worsening and thus increasing the likelihood of an underlying dementia.

What will happen to the generation who has grown up using digital clocks? Indeed, for them this test may become obsolete. However, in the meantime we still have many more years of the current cohort of middle-aged and elderly people for whom this test will still be useful (Shulman, 2018).

Mini-Cog

The Mini-Cog (Screening for Cognitive Impairment in Older Adults) combines clock-drawing with three-item recall, improving sensitivity compared to clock-drawing alone. It was developed to identify individuals with clinically important cognitive impairment in primary care settings. Verbal fluency (word generation) tests, in particular initial letter fluency, are also widely used as tests of executive dysfunction. Patients are asked to generate words from initial letters (normally F, A, and S or C, F, and L) and/or broad semantic categories (animals, fruits, or vegetables) under time constraints.

The Mini-Cog (Borson et al., 2000) is a very short test (3 min) suitable for primary care screening for dementia. It incorporates the clock-drawing test, adding a three-item delayed word recall task. It showed comparable sensitivity and specificity to the Mini Mental State Examination (MMSE) in classifying community cases of dementia (Borson et al., 2003).

MoCA

One of the most useful practical cognitive screening tools available to the geriatric forensic evaluator, the MoCA is in the public domain and also included as an Appendix at the end of this book. Unlike the Mini Mental State Exam (MMSE) or the Clock-Drawing Test (CDT), the MoCA is designed to detect more subtle impairments of cognition, known clinically as Mild Cognitive Impairment (MCI). Like the MMSE, it is scored out of 30, which can cause a misunderstanding about the severity of cognitive dysfunction for older adults.

The MOCA (Montreal Cognitive Assessment) was originally developed as a brief cognitive screening tool for detection of Mild Cognitive Impairment (MCI), but has since become widely used in clinical and research settings, often supplanting the MMSE. It consists of number of separate tasks covering 6 different cognitive domains including executive function skills. While not a substitute for in-depth neuropsychological testing, the MOCA correlates well with more comprehensive formal neuropsychological testing.

The MoCA is in the public domain. Evaluators can access the MoCA online at https://www.mocatest.org/

The Montreal Cognitive Assessment (Nasreddine et al., 2005) was originally developed to help screen for Mild Cognitive Impairment (MCI). It takes minimal training and can be used for about 10 min by any clinician. It assesses attention/concentration, executive functions, conceptual thinking, memory, language, calculation, and orientation. A score of 25 or lower (from maximum of 30) is considered significant cognitive impairment. It performs at least as well as MMSE, including in screening for dementia. It has been widely translated. As it assesses executive function, it is particularly useful for patients with vascular impairment, including vascular dementia (Sheehan, 2012).

It is not uncommon for a normally functioning older adult to score in the low 20s on the MoCA while the same individual can score high on the MMSE. In an individual with limited education and normal intelligence, a low score on the MoCA may represent a false positive result. However, the MoCA can pick up mild cognitive change in a highly intelligent and well-educated individual. Unlike the MMSE, it includes tests of higher-level brain function such as: abstract ability (similarities), verbal fluency (word generation with the phonemic prime of the letter 'F'), and it also includes the Clock-Drawing Test and a more difficult Delayed Memory Test. (Shulman, 2018).

To be of value, the MoCA needs to be interpreted in the context of a good history, appropriate investigations and importantly, what reliable informants say about an individual's functioning. It is especially valuable as a baseline to monitor cognitive change over time when the initial screen or assessment is equivocal with respect to a diagnosis of dementia.

A single score on the MoCA, is not diagnostic of dementia, and says very little about capacity per se.

MMSE

Clinicians and lawyers are regularly exposed to a score on the Mini Mental State Exam (MMSE) also known as the 'Folstein test' after the developer of the most widely used cognitive screening tool in the world. Yet it is one of the most misunderstood and misinterpreted tests in medicine. The popular MMSE (Mini Mental State Examination), the most-used assessment scale in dementia, does not assess executive function. The MMSE was primarily designed to test global cognitive function. It can be used to evaluate delirium or dementia, screen for global cognitive impairment, estimate the severity of cognitive impairment, and to follow changes in an individual over time. Patients can have a normal MMSE score despite executive function impairment with severe functional limitations. The MMSE is no longer in the public domain and may be too costly for some settings.

The MMSE (Folstein et al., 1975) is the best known and most widely used measure of cognition in clinical practice worldwide. This scale can be easily administered by clinicians or researchers with minimal training, takes around 10 min and assesses cognitive function in the areas of orientation, memory, attention and calculation, language and visual construction. Patients score between 0 and 30 points, and cutoffs of 23/24 have typically been used to show significant cognitive impairment. It is widely translated and used. A standardized version improves its reliability, and is probably most important for research settings.

The MMSE is unfortunately sometimes misunderstood as a diagnostic test, when it is in fact a screening test with relatively modest sensitivity. It has floor and ceiling effects and limited sensitivity to change. This in theory should limit its wider use in detecting change in clinical work and in research studies, though in these contexts it is still widely used, and even advocated (cite Sheehan, 2012).

The MMSE is a cognitive screening tool that provides a quick and easy method of assessing cognitive functioning. It is scored out of a possible 30 points and includes several cognitive domains including: Orientation to time and place, immediate and delayed recall, attention and concentration (spelling WORLD backwards or subtracting serial 7's from 100), as well as a visuo-spatial test (intersecting pentagons).

Over, the MMSE score can be used to provide a reasonably sensitive measure of cognitive change over time which in turn helps a clinician in conforming whether a progressive neurodegenerative disorder.

The MMSE is not in the public domain.

The MMSE will generally underestimate cognitive impairment when used head-to-head against the MoCA.

SLUMS

The SLUMS (St. Louis University Mental Status Examination) was created as a screening tool for detecting Mild Cognitive Impairment in a veteran population but is now used in several other patient populations (Morley and Tumosa, 2002). The SLUMS been shown to be superior to the Mini Mental State Exam (MMSE) in the detection of early dementia, and comparable to the popular Montreal Cognitive Assessment (MOCA).

Trail making tests A and B

The Trail Making Test (TMT) is an evaluation tool that has two parts that are referred to as the Trail Making Test Part A and the Trail Making Test Part B. It is a timed test and the goal is to complete the tests accurately and as quickly as possible.

The TMT Part A consists of 25 circles on a piece of paper with the numbers 1—25 written randomly in the circles. The test taker's task is to start with number one and draw a line from that circle to the circle with the number two in it to the circle with the three in it, etc. The TMT Part B consists of 24 circles on a piece of paper, but rather than all of the circles containing numbers, half of the circles have the numbers 1—12 in them and the other half (12) contain the letters A-L.

The Trail Making Test is scored by how long it takes to complete the test. The results of the TMT were found to be influenced significantly by age - as people age, they require a longer time to complete the TMT.

The TMT measures attention, visual screening ability, and processing speed, and is a good measure of overall cognitive functioning. Part A is a good measure of rote memory. Part B is generally quite sensitive to executive functioning since the test requires multiple abilities to complete it. The oral version of the TMT can be a quick tool to assess cognition when the person physically is unable to perform the written test or in situations like a hospital where illness and fatigue could affect the written results.

Pros and cons of the trails making test

Pros

- Free to use, while other tests require incur a cost each time they're administered
- Brief, taking only about 5 min to administer
- Part B has been shown to be a good measure of executive functioning. Tests that only measure memory or word-finding ability may miss impaired executive functioning and thus not detect some types of dementia.

Cons

- Older age generally affects performance, even in the absence of any cognitive impairment, but this is not taken into account in the scoring

CDR

The Clinical Dementia Rating scale allows more reliable staging of dementia than MMSE, and is based on caregiver accounts of problems in daily functional and cognitive tasks (Center, 2018). It takes only a few minutes for clinicians already familiar with individual cases, and classifies people with dementia into questionable, mild, moderate, and severe (Sheehan, 2012).

EXIT

The EXIT (Executive Interview) and Quick EXIT are screening instruments for executive cognitive dysfunction in patients with mild dementia, both designed to be administered at the bedside by non-neuropsychiatric ally trained personnel. EXIT scores correlate with neuropsychological and neuropsychiatric test batteries. They are simple to administer and use a single form as the only material required for the test, including instructions and scoring instructions. Executive function as measured by the EXIT25 is associated with multiple decision-making capacity domains (Schillerstrom et al., 2007).

FAB

The FAB (Frontal Assessment Battery) is a brief tool that can be used at the bedside or in a clinical setting to assist in assessing executive function and discriminating between cortical and subcortical dementias. It tests abstraction, fluency, impulsivity, and primitive reflexes. The FAB takes less than 10 min to administer and provides an objective measure to distinguish frontotemporal dementia from Alzheimer's disease in mildly demented patients. The study by Slachevsky et al. revealed that while the FAB was able to distinguish between the two diseases at early onset, the MMSE was not capable of doing so (Holzer et al., 2018).

Global deterioration scale

The Global Deterioration Scale (Reisberg et al., 1982) is essentially for staging dementia and takes only 2 min, once relevant clinical information has been collated. It has been well validated and classifies cases into seven stages from no complaints through to very severe. Like CDR, it is mainly used to assort cases by severity in research or in-service development, as in an individual case, more subtle changes which are important may not be picked up (Sheehan, 2012).

Strengths and drawbacks of selected screening tests

Test	Strengths	Further information
CLOX (Executive Clock Drawing Task), **CDT** (Clock Drawing Test)	Quick to administer (<5 min)	https://www.researchgate.net/publication/13684856_CLOX_An_executive_clock_drawing_task
Mini-Cog (Screening for Cognitive Impairment in Older Adults)	Quick to administer (<5 min)	https://mini-cog.com/http://www.ftdrg.org/wp-content/uploads/Test-Instructions.pdf
MOCA (Montreal Cognitive Assessment)	Quick to administer (15–20 min) Correlates with more comprehensive testing	http://www.mocatest.org/
SLUMS (St. Louis University Mental Status Examination)	Quick to administer (<15 min) Correlates with more comprehensive testing	https://www.slu.edu/medicine/internal-medicine/geriatric-medicine/aging-sucessfully/assessment-tools/mental-status-exam.php
Verbal fluency (word list generation)	Quick to administer (<5 min)	https://www.asha.org/Events/convention/handouts/2012/1527-The-3-Minute-

(*Continued*)

—cont'd

Test	Strengths	Further information
		Assessment-Clinical-Profiles-Associated-With-Verbal-Fluency/
FAB (Frontal Assessment Battery)	Quick to administer (<15 min)	https://www.meded.help/wp-content/uploads/2017/04/Frontal_FAB_Scale.pdf?x30812
EXIT25 (Executive Interview), **Quick EXIT**	Quick to administer (EXIT25 15–20 min, Quick EXIT 10 min)	https://www.researchgate.net/publication/21709157_Bedside_Assessment_of_Executive_Cognitive_Impairment_The_Executive_Interview
Formal neuropsychological testing (Wisconsin Card Sorting Test, Stroop Color-Word Interference Test, Trail Making Test, and others)	Gold standard, provides most detailed information Drawbacks: Time consuming (hours) Costly Difficult to access May not be well tolerated by patients with comorbid medical or psychiatric conditions	http://razlab.mcgill.ca/docs/cambridgehandbook_290.pdf

Test norms for older adults

The ethics code of the American Psychological Association advises psychologists to "make reasonable efforts to maintain the integrity and security of test materials and other assessment techniques consistent with law and contractual obligations… " Indicate whether the normative group differed in any significant ways from the evaluee. For example, if you are using a test that has been normed on young adults with an elderly evaluee, this fact should be noted as a limitation of the assessment.

Forensic psychiatrists occasionally conduct psychological testing, for a host of reasons that may include a lack of access to psychological consultation, a lack of funding for such consultation, or a genuine belief that they are technically and legally qualified to select, administer, score, and interpret the most suitable instruments for informing a particular medicolegal opinion.

This phenomenon may have several clinical, ethical, and legal ramifications, depending on the forensic psychiatrist's level of training, the forensic issues being addressed, and the nature of the psychological tests employed (Dattilio and Gutheil, 2011).

When to refer to a neuropsychologist

In more complex cases, or if further information is needed beyond what can reasonably be obtained in the constraints of the forensic examination, clinicians should consider referring to formal neuropsychological testing in order to further explore an elder's cognitive functioning capacities, in cases where the nature or extent of deficits is unclear. Geriatric forensic evaluators should understand the potential utility of neuropsychological assessments, and take the time to explore how to critically evaluate and interpret the neuropsychological findings regarding geriatric evaluations in a forensic setting.

Neuropsychological evaluation can assist with a common issue of capacity when dealing with elders. It is used to identify, localize and assess specific areas of neurocognitive dysfunction, including the major domains of cognition, language, memory, executive functions, visual spatial abilities, performance validity, and compare the data with normative samples to pick up individual patterns of cognitive strengths and weaknesses in a particular individual. This can assist in the diagnosis of cognitive disorders. It can also serve as a baseline for that individual's cognitive status should subsequent testing be required.

If the clinician is having trouble understanding elderly persons cognitive vulnerabilities, neuropsychological testing can help carefully assess the elder's strengths and weaknesses, as well as help with the identification of interventions or supports that may enhance their capacity and independence, or at least help identify restrictive accommodations to preserve an older person's dignity and autonomy.

Conclusion

In the older population, where cognitive difficulties can have a significant impact on mental functioning, the cognitive evaluation is particularly important in a geriatric forensic context. It can be challenging to initially apply a broad approach, select appropriate screening test, and then refine the assessment to provide a more detailed picture of what is relevant, particularly to a specific legal question being asked or standard being applied. For this purpose, multiple screening tests are available. In more complex cases, clinicians may want to consider referring the evaluee for formal neuropsychological testing.

Selected references

Agronin, M.E., 2014. Alzheimer's Disease and Other Dementias: A Practical Guide. Routledge, Taylor & Francis Group, New York.

American Psychiatric, A., American Psychiatric Association, D.S.M.T.F., 2013. Diagnostic and Statistical Manual of Mental Disorders: DSM-5. American Psychiatric Association, Arlington, Va.. Arlington, vol. a.

Borson, S., Scanlan, J., Chen, P., Ganguli, M., 2003. The Mini-Cog as a screen for dementia: validation in a population-based sample. J. Am. Geriatr. Soc. 51 (10), 1451−1454.

Boyle, P.A., Yu, L., Wilson, R.S., Gamble, K., Buchman, A.S., Bennett, D.A., 2012. Poor decision making is a consequence of cognitive decline among older persons without Alzheimer's disease or mild cognitive impairment. PLoS One 7 (8), e43647.

Center, K.A.S.D.R., 2018. CDR™ the Clinical Dementia Rating from. http://knightadrc.wustl.edu/cdr/cdr.htm.

Dattilio, F., Gutheil, T., 2011. Should forensic psychiatrists conduct psychological testing? Am. J. Psychiat. Law 39 (3), 477−491.

Edersheim, J., Murray, E.D., Padmanabhan, J.L., Price, B.H., 2017 Mar. Protecting the health and finances of the elderly with early cognitive impairment. J. Am. Acad. Psychiatry Law 45 (1), 81−91.

Folstein, M.F., Folstein, S.E., McHugh, P.R., 1975. "Mini-mental state" practical method for grading the cognitive state of patients for the clinician. J. Psychiatr. Res. 12 (3), 189−198.

Gibson, S. Forensic Interviewing with Older Adults. 2017. U.S. Department of Justice, Elder Justice Initiative. https://www.justice.gov/elderjustice/video/forensic-interviewing-older-adults

Granacher, 2018. Behavioral Neurological Aspects Involving the Elderly and the Law.

Han, S.D., Boyle, P.A., James, B.D., Yu, L., Bennett, D.A., 2016a. Mild cognitive impairment and susceptibility to scams in old age. J. Alzheimer's Dis. 49 (3), 845−851.

Han, S.D., Boyle, P.A., James, B.D., Yu, L., Barnes, L.L., Bennett, D.A., 2016b. Discrepancies between cognition and decision making in older adults. Aging Clin. Exp. Res. 28 (1), 99−108.

Holzer, J.C., Kohn, R., Ellison, J.M., Recupero, P.R., 2018. Geriatric Forensic Psychiatry: Principles and Practice. Oxford University Press, New York, NY.

Jack, C.R., Knopman, D.S., Jagust, W.J., Shaw, L.M., Aisen, P.S., Weiner, M.W., Petersen, R.C., Trojanowski, J.Q., 2010. Hypothetical model of dynamic biomarkers of the Alzheimer' s pathological cascade. Lancet Neurol. 9 (1), 119−128.

Jack Jr., C.R., Bennett, D.A., Blennow, K., Carrillo, M.C., Dunn, B., Haeberlein, S.B., Holtzman, D.M., Jagust, W., Jessen, F., Karlawish, J., Liu, E., Molinuevo, J.L., Montine, T., Phelps, C., Rankin, K.P., Rowe, C.C., Scheltens, P., Siemers, E., Snyder, H.M., Sperling, R., Contributors, 2018. NIA-AA Research Framework: toward a biological definition of Alzheimer's disease. Alzheimer's Dement. 14 (4), 535−562.

Mainland, B.J., Shulman, K.I., 2013. Clock drawing test. In: Cognitive Screening Instruments – A Practical Approach. Springer, pp. 79–109.
Morley, J., Tumosa, N., 2002. Saint Louis University mental status examination (SLUMS). Aging Successfully 12 (1), 4.
Nasreddine, Z.S., Phillips, N.A., Bedirian, V., et al., 2005. The Montreal Cognitive Assessment, MoCA: a brief screening tool for mild cognitive impairment. J. Am. Geriatr. Soc. 53 (4), 695–699.2.
Price, B.H., December 12, 2013. Decision making in mild cognitive impairment and Alzheimer's disease. In: Presentation, MGH Center for Law, Brain and Behavior and Boston Society for Neurology and Psychiatry. http://clbb.mgh.harvard.edu/capacity-finances-and-the-elderly-brain-science-meets-the-law/.
Reisberg, B., Ferris, S., De Leon, M., Crook, T., 1982. The Global Deterioration Scale for assessment of primary degenerative dementia. Am. J. Psychiatry 139 (9), 1136–1139.
Rosen, A., 2017. Neurocognitive Disorders of the DSM-5. Mental Illness Research, Education, and Clinical Center (MIRECC). VA Palo Alto Health Care System.
Rosenbloom, M., Schmahmann, J., Price, B., 2012. The functional neuroanatomy of decision-making. J. Neuropsychiatry Clin. Neurosci. 24 (3), 266–277.
Royall, D.R., Cordes, J.A., Polk, M.C.L.O.X., 1998. An executive clock drawing task. J. Neurol. Neurosurg. Psychiatry 64, 588–594.
Sachdev, P.S., Blacker, D., Blazer, D.G., Ganguli, M., Jeste, D.V., Paulsen, J.S., Petersen, R.C., 2014. Classifying neurocognitive disorders: the DSM-5 approach. Nat. Rev. Neurol. 10 (11), 634–642.
Schillerstrom, J.E., Rickenbacker, D., Joshi, K.G., Royall, D.R., 2007. Executive function and capacity to consent to a noninvasive research protocol. Am. J. Geriatr. Psychiatry 15 (2), 159–162.
Sheehan, B., 2012. Assessment scales in dementia. Ther. Adv. Neurol. Disord. 5, 349–358.
Shulman, K., 2018. All about Estates – Blog Posts 2014-2016 from. https://www.allaboutestates.ca/author/kshulman/.
Shulman, K.I., Hull, I.M., DeKoven, S., Amodeo, S., Mainland, B.J., Herrmann, N., 2015. Cognitive fluctuations and the lucid interval in dementia: implications for testamentary capacity. J. Am. Acad. Psychiat. Law 43 (3), 287–292.
Simpson, J.R., 2014. DSM-5 and neurocognitive disorders. J. Am. Acad. Psychiat. Law 42 (2), 159–164.
Squire, L.R., 1987. Memory and Brain. Oxford University Press, Oxford, UK.
Verdelho, A., Gonçalves-Pereira, M., 2016. Neuropsychiatric Symptoms of Cognitive Impairment and Dementia. Springer International Publishing.
Weintraub, S., Randolph, C., Bain, L., Hendrix, J.A., Carrillo, M.C., 2017. Is cognitive decline measurable in preclinical Alzheimer's disease? Alzheimers Dement 13 (3), 322–323. https://doi.org/10.1016/j.jalz.2017.02.002.

CHAPTER FOUR

Evaluation of decision-making capacity and guardianship

Contents

The Clinician's Guide to Geriatric Forensic Evaluations
ISBN: 978-0-12-815034-4
https://doi.org/10.1016/B978-0-12-815034-4.00004-0

A 90-year-old widower was living on his own despite memory and cognitive problems. His wife died a few years earlier, and he had no family in the region. His out-of-state relatives telephoned him regularly to check in. The relatives became concerned after a married couple approached the widower offering to help, and initially the widower and relatives welcomed their assistance to help him around the house and perform minor home repairs. However, soon the couple had taken over supervising his care, controlling his money, and restricting his access to his family.

Decision-making capacity is a dominant issue in forensic geriatric psychiatry given the increasing prevalence of cognitive impairment with aging and other factors fostering dependency in older people. Cognitive and functional losses in individuals with dementia often coincide with losses in decision-making capacity, including the capacity to consent to medical treatment, treatment and the management of everyday functional abilities, such as managing finances. Losses in decision-making capacity may lead to guardianship petitions, questions of capacity to consent to medical treatment, the ability to make a new will, or participate in human research.

In seeking to resolve these issues, families, clinicians, and legal professionals increasingly turn to psychiatrists, psychologists, and other mental health professionals to assess capacity, and help the courts properly balance autonomy and protection for the individual (Moye, Marson et al., 2013b). None of the usual areas of clinical focus - including diagnosis, mental status findings, cognitive function, rapport - are the sole basis for decision making capacity, though they can certainly inform the clinician's overall assessment. Instead, is important to remember that capacity is task- and domain-specific, so that incapable in one area does not necessarily mean incapable in others.

Principles of capacity assessment

Capacity is a medico-legal construct. In this chapter, capacity and competence or competency will be considered to be equivalent terms, reflecting common usage in medical settings and the terms capacity and competence are often used interchangably. However, in strictly proper usage capacity applies in the clinical setting and competency resides in the purview of the court.

Strict definitions: capacity versus competence

- Capacity – clinical setting
- Competence – purview of the court

Concerns about decision-making capacity can arise from clinical, ethical, and medicolegal perspectives. Clinicians are confronted with many questions about assessing older adults for decision-making capacity. Questions include who to talk to before the assessment, determining whether an attorney is involved, understanding the definition of lack of capacity, the role of family, the forensic report, use of cognitive testing, objective capacity measures and instruments, and other technical questions. Clinicians may also wonder how to approach the patient, taking into account the patient's history and values in decision making and the final capacity judgment. Finally, clinicians will want to consider how to phrase their findings so they will be understandable to the court (ABA/APA, 2008, p. 8).

Framework for capacity assessment

It is helpful to have a framework of the most important elements in assessment of decision-making capacity to guide the evaluation process. The framework below is based on the 9-part model outlined in the ABA/APA guide to Assessment of Older Adults with Diminished Capacity (2008), which is an expansion of psychologist Tom Grisso's pinoeering model for legal capacity (1986) that originally included six of the elements. This 9-part model expands on Grisso's framework for the context of clinical assessment of decision-making capacity and need for guardianship in older adults.

9-part framework for capacity assessment

- Identify the applicable legal standard(s)
- Identify and evaluating functional elements constituent to the capacity
- Determine relevant medical and psychiatric diagnoses contributing to incapacity
- Evaluate cognitive functioning
- Consider psychiatric and/or emotional factors
- Appreciate the individual's values
- Identify risks related to the individual and situation
- Consider means to enhance the individual's capacity
- Make a clinical judgment of capacity

ABA/APA, 2008; Grosso, 1986

Functional capacity

Functional capacity refers to specific behavioral tasks and cognitive decision-making required for a specific capacity domain. For example, functional capacity may include the ability to provide self-care i.e. provide oneself with food, clothing, shelter, and medical care, and manage one's finances. Functional capacity involves executive functioning and complex decision making, including elements of motivation, prioritization, planning, and execution of goal-oriented sequences of behavior over time (Holzer et al., 2018).

Functional assessment for the purpose of capacity evaluation is closely tied with legal definitions of capacity (ABA/APA, 2008). Functional capacity can be assessed through formal means such as structured testing, or by informal means, such as observing the individual and asking the individual, family and staff questions.

Binary, dichotomous capacity decisions versus concept of marginal capacity

In most situations, geriatric forensic evaluators are expected to arrive at a "binary" or "dichotomous" answer to the specific capacity question. However, in many situations, capacity may be operating as more of a continuous variable. Integration of data to arrive at a dichotomous conclusion can be a new and uncomfortable role for the clinician evaluator tasked with considering all the data and offering an opinion about whether the data, considered in context, leans more in favor of or against the person's capacity. It may help to further delineate the capacity task—e.g., the person has the capacity to make a simple medical decision but not a complex or high-risk one.

At times, clinicians may not be able to provide a strict "yes or no" answer. In such cases a clinician may say the person has marginal capacity. A finding of "marginal capacity" rather than a yes/no finding, does not necessarily represent discomfort with "sticking one's neck out" and offering a clear opinion.

The image below visually depicts the tension between clinical notions of decision-making capacity, and the yes-no clarity of a court's capacity judgment. Clinicians are often caught in this tension and should keep in mind the concept of marginal decision-making capacity (ABA/APA, 2008).

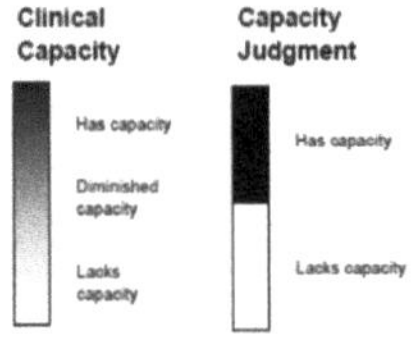

From ABA/APA Assessment of Capacity in Older Adults Project Working Group., American Bar Association. Commission on Law and Aging. and American Psychological Association. (2008). Assessment of older adults with diminished capacity: a handbook for psychologists. Washington, D.C., American Bar Association Commission on Law and Aging: American Psychological Association. Copyright © 2008 American Bar Association and American Psychological Association. Reproduced with permission.

Definition of capacity/competence

Appelbaum and Grisso (Appelbaum and Grisso, 1988) delineated four components of decisional capacity in the medical setting: the ability to (1) communicate effectively, (2) understand relevant information, (3) appreciate the situation and its consequences, and (4) rationally manipulate information. These concepts have become the most consistently accepted framework regarding consent to medical care.

Appelbaum and Grisso's 4 basic abilties of decisional capacity

- Communicate effectively
- Understand relevant information
- Appreciate the situation and its consequences
- Rationally manipulate information (Appelbaum and Grisso, 1988).

In every case, there is a presumption of capacity.

Presume capacity until proven otherwise

Routine capacity screening of whole classes of individuals cannot and should not be endorsed, as this prejudges an individual's capacity based on class membership. For example, it is incorrect to assume that all intellectually disabled persons must be incapable by virtue of their disability. It is incorrect to assume that a diagnosis of a severe psychiatric disorder like schizophrenia renders the person unable to meet his or her personal care or financial needs.

There should be reasonable grounds that prompt the request for a formal capacity assessment.

Even a severe mental disorder like dementia or schizophrenia does not necessarily render a person unable to meet certain personal care or financial needs.

Concerns about decision-making capacity can arise from clinical, ethical, and medical and legal perspectives. An assessment of decision-making capacity refers to a specific and particular situation. An illness may cause impairment of mental functions or reveal the presence and consequences of pre-existing cognitive impairment. Questions may arise among care providers from family or friends about decision-making capacity and other domains, such as finance, personal relations, or business.

Clinicans should always endeavor to consider the specifics of the laws and statutes relevant to a particular case. Thankfully, considerable overlap is found among most states on these issues.

Capacity is task-specific and domain-specific

For many older adults with diminished capacity, the notion of global incapacity is problematic. Current thinking about decision-making capacity is that incapacity is domain-specific. Decision-making capacity may be limited only with respect to certain decisions or classes of decisions.

As in all of medicine, diagnosis and clinical (and legal) determinations about decision-making capacity depend on multiple factors. Decision-making capacity is almost never determined by a single score on the MMSE (except perhaps in extremely low scores). Moreover, capacity is not determined solely by the presence of dementia. An older adult can be cognitively impaired yet potentially maintain the capacity make decisions, depending on their complexity.

Capacity is not determined by dementia or by screening test score.

The ability to examine decision-making in a more circumscribed fashion ensures that the person's rights will not be removed in areas where he or she is still able to manage.

Capacity for decision-making does not need to be formally examined in areas where there are no presenting concerns. For example, a person may have severe dementia that precludes his or her ability to meet essential personal care needs, but if the individual is already in safe housing, he or she may only require a capacity assessment for property (Ontario, 2010).

When you receive a request for a capacity assessment, the first question to ask is: Capacity for what?

Capacity is domain-specific

At the broadest level, the law can recognize that a person may lack capacity in one area but not the other. For example, it can distinguish between the ability to make financial and personal care decisions, and those ca can further be subdivided into banking, contracts, health care, nutrition, clothing, hygiene, shelter, safety, etc. Capacity can be independently assessed in any, several or all of these sub-domains, and the assessor could find the person incapable in one or more or all.

Principle of proportionality

To expand on Appelbaum and Grisso's 4 abilities concept, in every case, as the complexity of the situation and the number of available options increases, the mental ability required to make a competent decision also increases.

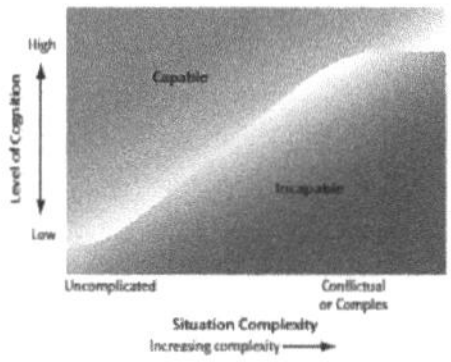

From Shulman, K. I., C. A. Cohen, F. C. Kirsh, I. M. Hull and P. R. Champine (2007). "Assessment of testamentary capacity and vulnerability to undue influence." American Journal of Psychiatry 164(5): 722–727. Reprinted with permission from American Journal of Psychiatry, (Copyright © 2007). American Psychiatric Association. All Rights Reserved.

According to this principle of proportionality, the depth of ability that the patient must demonstrate for the clinician to conclude that the patient retains capacity depends on the benefit/risk ratio of the proposed decision. For example, administration of glucose for insulin induced hypoglycemia or IV hydration, interventions with very high benefit and very little risk, would require only basic understanding and appreciation of the risks and benefits to be judged as having capacity. On the other hand, consenting to an invasive and risky procedure like surgical resection of a brain lesion, or going home alone without support services that are adequate, would require a much more sophisticated understanding of the risks, benefits, and alternative approaches (Roth et al., 1977).

Clinicians may find themselves in situations where persuasion can be considered ethical, such as in the context of an established doctor-patient relationship with rapport which may at times be used to help a patient accept treatment for medical condition which would reasonably be expected to improve their condition. However, coercion is to be avoided since it would result in an involuntary consent (Buchanan, 2004).

Components of informed consent

- the nature and seriousness of the illness, disorder, or defect that the person has
- the nature of the medical treatment that is being recommended by the person's health care providers
- the probable degree and duration of any benefits and risks of any medical intervention that is being recommended by the person's health care providers, and the consequences of lack of treatment
- the nature, risks, and benefits of any reasonable alternatives

Holzer et al., 2018

Cognitive ability is the most consistent correlate of decisional capacity. Scores on tests of cognitive function, including assessment of executive functions, can predict functional impairment and dementia (Chen et al., 1998). The use of standardized tests of cognition is recommended, but it is important to use caution in interpretation of screening test results. Historical evidence from collateral sources regarding relevant abilities and functions of findings from neuropsychological testing should be considered.

The expert who relies on DSM-5 categories for neurocognitive disorders should be prepared to explain how this new terminology relates to the term dementia, while anticipating the possibility a line of attack on terminological arbitrariness (Simpson, 2014).

A collaborative approach

The capacity to execute a will, power of Attorney (POA), manage property, personal care or marry are cognitive tasks determined by an admixture of legal, statutory, and clinical guidelines and factors.

Multiple resources are available to assist practitioners with identifying common ethical issues and challenges. Experienced colleagues often serve as one of the richest sources of information, as the experiences and advice of senior colleagues provide one important perspective to help clinicians anticipate, avoid, and address ethical challenges (Bush et al., 2015). Capacity to make decisions such as execute a will, power of Attorney (POA), manage property, personal care or marry, are cognitive tasks determined by an a mixture of legal, statutory, and clinical guidelines and factors.

Personal values and emotional factors in decision making

Traditional cognitive views of decision-making competence err in not taking into account patient's emotional capacities. There may be stronger arguments for broadening the focus of competence assessment to include emotional capacities, centering on the ways in which emotions aid humans in processing information (Appelbaum, 1998). Instruments and resources for assessing patient values include an advance directive called "Five wishes", the Values and Preferences Scale (VPS), and other self report measures for values assessment (ABA/APA, 2008). Personal and personality factors influencing decision-making are listed in the table below.

An individual's decision about medical care can be influenced by many factors including cultural background, religious beliefs, personal priorities, prior experiences with illness and care systems, and economics. Aging itself has also been shown to affect processing and retention of information provided during the capacity and consent process. Some personal and personality factors affecting medical decision making are listed below.

Personal and personality factors affecting medical decision-making

- Education may affect comprehension of information necessary for decision-making
- Lifelong avoidance of doctors, medications
- May resist acknowledging need for medical invention
- Previous bad medical experience or outcome for self or family member
- May distrust medical providers
- Strong religious beliefs: depending on religion, may adhere to doctrine regarding advance directives, withdrawal of care
- Limited financial resources
- May not believe that necessary care is affordable
- Responsibility for another family member: may believe that accepting medical care will interfere with caregiving responsibilities.

Holzer et al., (2018)

Assessors should be aware of possible differences in values between themselves and older people individuals they assess. They should be careful not to make value judgments based on their experiences and keep in mind that older people may have experienced different things in their lifetime.

Evaluators should try to understand the natural fears of older people — for example, the fear of losing their independence and their home.

Ageism and myths about decision-making capacity

Evaluators should beware of ageist attitudes that may bias them in their assessment about decision-making capacity. Remember that age itself, does not determine capacity. Very elderly persons can be completely capable of making all decisions on their own behalf. Clinicians should be aware of possible differences in values between themselves and older people individuals they assess. Evaluators should take care not to make value judgments based on their own experience, and should keep in mind that older people may have experienced different things in their lifetime.

Ten myths about capacity

1. Decision-making capacity = competency
2. Against medical advice = lack of decision-making capacity
3. There's no need to assess decision-making capacity unless a patient goes against medical advice
4. Decision-making capacity is all or nothing
5. Cognitive impairment = no decision-making capacity
6. Lack of decision-making capacity is permanent
7. Patients who have not been given relevant information about their condition can lack decision-making capacity
8. All patients with certain psychiatric disorders lack decision-making capacity
9. All institutionalized patients lack decision-making capacity
10. Only psychiatrists and psychologists can assess decision-making capacity

Ganzini et al., 2004

Types of decision-making capacity

This section will explore key areas of decision-making capacity that may a focus of geriatric forensic evaluations. Where available, sections below will include ways to maximize capacity in older people, i.e. a wide range of legal and social interventions that can be used to assist someone with functional or decisional compromise instead of guardianship.

Capacity to make medical decisions

92-year-old Mrs. G is admitted to the hospital after she called 911 because of back pain. On the medical service, she is treated with pain medications and referred to skilled nursing facility for additional therapy and pain management. Mrs. G refuses and says she wants to go home. Staff is concerned that she has risk of falling.

Holzer et al, 2018

There is a large array of different tasks and functions a consulting psychiatrist may be called upon to help with assessment and management, including end-of-life decision-making, assessing testamentary capacity, assisting family and conflict around end-of-life decisions and issues, pain relief and psychopharmacological management, agitation and aggression, and optimizing independence. Each of these domains can have important medical legal implications.

In the hospital setting, questions of capacity assessment regarding health-care decisions are only the beginning, and each request to assess the capacity and/or abilities of an elderly hospitalized patient presents unique challenges. Requests for an evaluation of medical decision-making capacity may lead to other questions like capacity to manage finances, requiring assessment of the ability to manage financial tasks, and understanding the scope of assets and expenses.

For medical decisions, including the right to accept or refuse treatment, the consulting clinician can engage questions of decisional capacity through a comprehensive approach that assesses for reversible medical conditions, develops an appreciation for the patient as a person, and ensures that the patient question has been adequately informed (Grisso and Appelbaum, 1998).

A variety of psychological and medical conditions can be responsible for impacting an older person's capacity to make medical and other decisions. Often, multiple etiologies are simultaneously involved. The table below summarizes common considerations for clinicians evaluating psychological or medical conditions potentially impacting capacity.

Psychological or medical conditions that can impact capacity, and measures to address them

- **Alcohol or other substances intoxication** - detoxification; supplement diet or another intake needs
- **Altered blood pressure** - treat underlying cause of blood pressure anomaly with medication or other treatment
- **Altered low blood sugar** - management of blood sugar through diet or medication
- **Anxiety** - treatment with medications and/or psychotherapy; support groups
- **Bereavement, recent death of a spouse or loved one** - support; counseling by therapist or clergy; support group; medications to assist in short-term problems (e.g. sleep, depression)
- **Bipolar disorder** - treatment with medications and/or psychotherapy; support groups
- **Brain tumor** - medical treatment as indicated, such as surgery, radiation, and medication
- **Delirium** - obtain standard labs; obtain brain scan if indicated; assess vitals; treat underlying cause; monitor and reassess over time
- **Dementia** - treatment with medications for dementia; simplify environment; provide multiple clues within environment; use step-by-step communication
- **Depression** - treatment with medications and/or psychotherapy; add pleasurable activities to day; ECT if indicated; support groups
- **Developmental disability** - education and training
- **Head injury** - treatments for acute effects (e.g., bleed, pressure, swelling) as necessary; monitoring over time; rehabilitative speech, physical, occupational therapies

(Continued)

Psychological or medical conditions that can impact capacity, and measures to address them (*cont'd*)

- **Infection** (e.g., urinary, influenza, pneumonia, meningitis) - treat underlying infection with antibiotic or other treatment
- **Insomnia** - sleep hygiene practices (e.g., limit caffeine, light exercise, limit naps); medications
- **Liver or kidney disease** - treatment of underlying illness with medication, dialysis, surgery.
- **Loneliness** - social and recreational activities; support groups
- **Malnutrition or dehydration** - IV fluids; fluid/food by mouth; food supplements; possible food by feeding tube
- **Mania** - treatment with medications and/or psychotherapy; support groups
- **Medications and sudden medication withdrawal** - review of medications by clinical pharmacist or specialist; slow one-by-one tapers or changes of medications
- **Poor heart or lung function (e.g. hypoxia)** - treatment of underlying condition with medication, surgery, supplemental oxygen
- **Post-surgical confusion** (usually related to anesthesia or pain medicines) - monitoring and reassessment over time; try alternative medications and treatments for pain management
- **Depression and anxiety** - psychotherapy, support, counseling by therapist or clergy; support group; medications to treat symptoms
- **Schizophrenia, hallucinations, or delusions** - treatment with medications for schizophrenia; simplify environment; provide support
- **Transfer trauma** (a recent move that has the individual disoriented) - monitoring over time; re-orientation to environment

Adapted from ABA/APA Guide, Professor Joan O'Sullivan (University of Maryland School of Law).

Advance directives

An 85-year-old woman suffered a massive stroke that rendered her unable to either speak or swallow independently. She received a feeding tube two years ago. Her guardian is now petitioning the court to remove the feeding tube, citing the patient's written advance directive.

An advance health care directive is a legal instrument intended to ensure that decisions regarding a person's medical care, made at such time as he or she becomes incompetent to give informed consent, will reflect the values and instructions made while the patient retains capacity.

There are generally two types of advance directives: proxy directives, such as the durable power of attorney for health care, and instruction directives, such as the living will. Proxy directives allow an individual, the principal, to authorize another person, most commonly a family member or spouse, the attorney-in-fact or agent, to give or withhold consent for medical care for the principle if the principal becomes incompetent.

With a durable power of attorney, a person known as the principal designates another to be his or her agent at a potentially future time if the principal becomes disabled or incapacitated in terms of decision-making.

A living will is a document that specifies the limits of care to be given by the healthcare providers of the individual determined to lose decisional capacity. Multiple topics may be addressed including treatments that the principal does not want, preferences regarding treatment at the end of his or her life, like the preference to be at home, and instructions regarding organ donation or autopsy. Some states also authorize inclusion of preferences for the disposal of remains.

With regards to advance directives for psychiatric decisions, some authors maintain that the capacity to make an advance directive is higher than that required to make a contemporaneous treatment decision. Unlike the assessment of contemporaneous capacity, it is very difficult to determine a person's capacity retrospectively or to determine if an advance directive was meant to apply in changed circumstances. If an advance directive demands a course of action that is contrary to a person's best interests, the onus may fall on the person rejecting the care to demonstrate that he or she was capable when executing the directive and that the directive is meant to apply in the current circumstances (O'Reilly, 2008).

If the person needs medical treatment, but is not able to consent

- Health Care Advance Directive: any written statement a competent individual has made concerning future health care decisions. The two typical forms of advance directive are the living will and the health care power of attorney
- Surrogate decision making by an authorized legal representative, a relative, or a close friend: in many states, the next of kin are authorized to make some or all medical treatment decisions in the absence of a health care advance directive or appointed guardian

Adapted from ABA/APA Guide, Professor Joan O'Sullivan (University of Maryland School of Law).

Capacity to appoint a health care proxy

It is important to weigh patients' understanding and choice within the context of the risks and benefits of the medical and interpersonal factors (Moye, Sabatino et al., 2013a). The appointment of a healthcare proxy is the most common way through which patients appoint a surrogate decision-maker in anticipation of a future time in which they may lack the ability to make medical decisions themselves. In some situations, if a patient has not previously appointed a surrogate decision-maker through an advance directive, the healthcare team may ask whether the patient, although lacking the capacity to make a healthcare decision, might still have the capacity to appoint a healthcare proxy.

If a patient is hospitalized without a designated surrogate decision-maker, states have legislation describing the hierarchy for selecting a default surrogate decision-maker for the incapacitated patient. A typical hierarchy is illustrated below.

Hierarchy of surrogate decision-makers in the absence of an advance directive

- Legal guardian
- Spouse
- Adult son or daughter
- Parent
- Adult sibling
- Adult grandchild or other adult relative who has been involved
- Close friend
- Guardian of the patient's estate

Holzer et al., 2018

Capacity to consent to research

Investigators generally address the ethical dilemma of patients' decisional impairment in Alzheimer disease (AD) research by obtaining consent from alternative or surrogate decision makers ("proxies") as well as assent from patients (Overton et al., 2013). Ethical guidelines suggest that, when enrolling patients with dementia in research, alterative decision makers (proxies) should base their decision on a "substituted judgment" of how the patient would have decided. If unable to make a substituted judgment, proxies are asked to decide on the basis of the patient's best interests (Dunn et al., 2013).

Capacity to live independently

Capacity or competency to go home, is a common question that consulting psychiatrist are asked to assess as well as inpatient medical setting. It includes the functional capacity to perform those tasks necessary to live at home safely, and also the decisional capacity to make a capable decision about going home, based on the available data.

There are many questions a clinician can ask to specifically determine an older person's capacity to live independently. These include questions about the living environment, visitors, family and community, and changes in the older person's functioning abilities. The text box below summarizes many of the questions to add to a clinical interview that specifically focus on issues relevant to the capacity to live independently.

Requisite capacities to live at home safely

- Safe mobility and transfers
- Communication
- Food and fluid
- Medication and medical management
- Money management

Holzer et al., 2018

Questions relevant to the capacity to live independently

- Where are you living now? How long have you been there?
- Does anyone live there with you? If not, do you have any fears or concerns about living alone?
- Does anyone visit on a regular basis?
- What family and/or friends live in your community who are important to you?
- What is most important to you about where you live? What makes it "home"?
- What kind of personal activities do you enjoy doing at home?
- Are there community activities in which you enjoy participating?

(Continued)

Questions relevant to the capacity to live independently (*cont'd*)

- What do you like about your house/apartment?
- What do you not like about your house/apartment? What does not work well for you and why?
- Do you feel that you can manage the house/apartment on your own? Have you noticed any changes in your abilities to manage?
- Are there areas of your life that you feel you may need some assistance managing? For instance, do you have any trouble with housekeeping, yard work, preparing meals, shopping, driving, using the telephone, the mail, your health, taking medications, managing your money, or paying bills on your own?
- Is there someone helping you with any of these things? If so, how long have they been assisting you?
- If you needed help, who would you like to help you? Is there anyone that you would be wary of? Why?
- Have you had any safety concerns at home? For instance, have you ever accidently left the stove or oven on, fallen and been unable to get up by yourself, left your doors unlocked, or invited a stranger into your home?
- Where would you like to live in the future?
- Have you ever considered moving to a place where there would be more help for you, such as senior housing, assisted living, or a nursing home? How do you feel about that? What fears or concerns do you have?

ABA/APA, 2008

Assessing the capacity of patients to make decisions about their functional problems, including the capacity to live independently, has substantial ethical, clinical, and financial implications. The growing population of older adults with cognitive impairment, either in the community or in long-term care and medical facilities, increase the importance of adequately assessing this capacity (Lai and Karlawish, 2007). Key features of capacity to live at home safely are listed below. These may be evaluated by a multidisciplinary team using different tests. Additional text boxes below include information options to consider if a person is living in an unsafe environment and needs help or supervision with activities of daily living.

Options for older adults living in an unsafe environment

Adapted from ABA/APA Guide, Professor Joan O'Sullivan (University of Maryland School of Law)

- **Senior shared housing programs** - several people live together in a group home or apartment with shared common areas. Personal care and health oversight are usually not part of services, but they may be provided through other community social services.
- **Adult foster care** - an older person who is in need of a modest amount of daily assistance is placed into a family home. The cost varies and may be covered in part by the state social services program.
- **Community residential care** - small supportive housing facilities that provide a room, meals, help with activities of daily living, and protective supervision to individuals who cannot live independently, but who do not need institutional care.
- **Assisted living** - facilities provide an apartment, meals, help with activities of daily living, and supervision to individuals who cannot live independently, but who do not need institutional care.
- **Nursing home** - skilled nursing care and services for residents who require medical or nursing care; or rehabilitation services for injured, disabled, or sick persons.
- **Continuing Care Retirement Communities (CCRCs)** - also called life care communities, these usually require the payment of a large entry fee, plus monthly fees thereafter. The facility may include options for independent living, assisted living, and nursing care. Residents move from one housing choice to another as their needs change.

Options for an older person needing help with activities of daily living or supervision

- **Care management** - A social worker or health care professional evaluates, plans, locates, coordinates, and monitors services for an older person and the family.
- **Home health services** - A visiting nurse or home health aide from a home health agency provides medical care or professional therapy on a part-time or intermittent basis
- **Home care services** - Homemaker or chore services can provide help with housework, laundry, ironing, and cooking. Personal care attendants or personal assistants may assist an impaired person in performing activities of daily living, (i.e., eating, dressing, bathing, toileting, and transferring), or with other activities instrumental to daily functioning.
- **Adult day care services** - Community-based group programs designed to meet the needs of functionally and/or cognitively impaired adults through an individual plan of care. Health, social, and other related support services are provided in a structured, protective setting.

(Continued)

Options for older adults living in an unsafe environment (*cont'd*)

- **Respite care programs** - Temporary care provided to people with disabilities so that their families can take a break from the daily routine of caregiving.
- **Meals on Wheels** - Volunteers deliver nutritious lunchtime meals to the homes of people who can no longer prepare balanced meals for themselves.
- **Transportation services** - Volunteers drive clients to and from medical, dental, or other necessary appointments, and remain with them throughout the visit.
- **Food and prescription drug deliveries** - Volunteer-based or commercially-based delivery services for food or prescription drugs, may assist those who are unable to leave their home regularly.
- **Medication reminder systems** - May include a weekly pill organizer box, or another pill distribution system, or telephone reminder calls.
- **Telephone reassurance programs** - Volunteers provide a daily telephone call to older persons living alone.
- **Home visitors and pets on wheels** - Elder service agencies and other volunteer agencies may match elders with home visitors, including visiting pets, which provide social interaction and a form of monitoring.
- **Daily checks on the person by mail carriers** - Many mail carriers, if notified that an elder at risk is living at an address, will monitor the home to ensure that mail has been picked up daily, and if not, notify a designated individual.
- **Housing modification** - To enhance safety and the use of technology in the home; grab bars, ramps, night wandering alarms, medication prompt systems, and home-telehealth monitors may be added.

In most states, there is unlikely to be a specific standard for "the capacity to live independently." Instead, the most relevant legal standards for the capacity to live independently are likely those which are defined in guardianship law. State statutes for incapacity under guardianship vary widely, but that many cite one or more of four "tests": the presence of a disabling condition; a functional element—sometimes defined as the inability to meet essential needs to live independently; a problem with cognition; and a necessity component, i.e. less restrictive alternatives to guardianship have failed *(ABA/APA 2008)*. The text box below summarizes APS statutes that have a "function" criterion, and their possible subcategories.

APS statutes with a "function" criterion:

- Lacking the ability to make, communicate, or implement decisions.
- Lacking the ability to understand the risks and consequences of behavior.
- Being dependent on others.
- Requiring care, treatment, or custody for own welfare or welfare of others.
- Restricted ability to carry out ADLs.
- Unable to care for or manage ones' self or property.
- Unable to delegate responsibility.
- Unable to perform or obtain services.
- Unable to protect self.

ABA/APA, 2008

Driving

Driving a motor vehicle is the preferred mode of transportation for the majority of older adults in the United States today. In addition to offering convenience, driving-based mobility supports personal autonomy and in- dependence, improved quality of life, and enhanced self-efficacy in comparison to non-drivers. As a group, older adults face unique risks as both drivers and passengers simply because of increased fragility. While the majority of older adults are capable drivers, some may be unfit due to medical-functional compromise. The prevention of death and serious injury is a primary goal, and a preventative-care approach is achievable. Such an approach involves viewing driving as a key instrumental activity of daily living (IADL) and thus a target for medical-functional assessment. Notably, many older drivers show concern and insight into driving habits and self-regulate by driving only during the daytime, driving slower, or limiting driving to shorter or non-highway distances. Actively involving the elderly adult in planning for future driving limitations and cessation may help to reduce the negative effects that a sudden and mandatory loss of driving privilege could have. For more information on advance care planning for driving changes see the Alzheimer's Association Web site at: http://www.alz.org/living_with_-alzheimers_driving.asp.

AGS Clinician's Guide to Assessing and Counseling Older Drivers

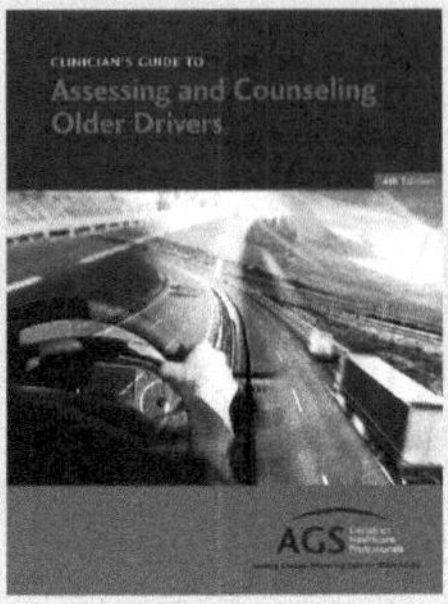

From AGS Clinician's guide to assessing and counseling older drivers, 4th edition (2019). Used with permission from the American Geriatrics Society.

The most important clinical resource for driving is the American Geriatrics Society's Clinician's guide to assessing and counseling older drivers, fourth edition (Pomidor, 2019). Highlights of this resource include preventive strategies, assessment and counseling techniques for clinicians to help them better identify older drivers at risk, enhance driving safety, and ease the transition to driving retirement when necessary.

Capacity to work, fitness for duty evaluations

Clinical and forensic fitness for duty evaluations are used to assess whether individuals are able to perform essential mental job functions of their positions with or without reasonable accommodations. FDE's are typically requested in response to specific incidents or complaints that raise suspicion of impairment, at times linked to issues of aging (Gold and Vanderpool, 2013). Detailed techniques of fitness for duty evaluations are beyond the scope of this volume, but they depend on the specific profession in question. Clinicians dealing with fitness for duty evaluations are advised to consult with relevant professional boards and licensing agencies as appropriate.

Capacity to vote

The right to vote can be abrogated when individuals become incompetent to cast a ballot. This applies particularly to people with Alzheimer's disease, who at some point will lose capacity.

The capacity to vote can be measured using a structured assessment that is particularly likely to be useful for people with moderate Alzheimer's disease, whose performance cannot be predicted from MMSE scores alone. This approach can ensure retention of voting rights by capable and exclusion of clearly impaired individuals from the voting booth (Appelbaum et al., 2005).

Sexual consent

An 81 year old man was charged with felony sexual abuse in relation to an incident where he allegedly had sexual contact with his wife at her nursing home. Prior to the incident, his wife's daughters from a previous marriage had met with nursing home staff, who advised the man that his wife no longer had the mental capacity to consent to sex.

Many clinicians hold negative attitudes toward sexual expression in late life, but sexual capacity is an important question, especially in the context of nursing homes. There is increased incidence of STDs at nursing homes and assisted living facilitie and sexual questions among older people have many unique aspects that are relatively understudied - for example, it may be difficult to convince a World War II veteran to use a condom.

Nursing home staffs' knowledge of sexuality and dementia, desire for guidance in "managing" sexual expression, and neutral attitudes toward late-life sexuality supports the need for educational interventions on sexuality and dementia in nursing homes (Di Napoli, Breland et al., 2013).

There are no universally accepted criteria for capacity to consent to sexual relations and the legal standards and criteria for sexual consent vary across states. The most widely accepted criteria, consistent with those applied to consent to medical treatment, are listed in the text box below.

Legal standard for sexual consent

- knowledge of relevant information, including risks and benefits
- understanding or rational reasoning that reveals a decision that is consistent with the individual's values (competence); and
- voluntariness (a stated choice without coercion)

ABA/APA, 2008

Committee decision-making for sexual expression, while it may seem like somewhat of a bizarre and frankly intrusive measure, may at least allow for continued discussion of the right to sexual freedom for a resident in the face of significant counterbalancing forces in the form of ageist stereotypes, risk of liability for a nursing home, and an overly medicalized approach to capacity assessments (Wilkins, 2016).

Sexual expression is an important aspect of well-being of older adults living in the community and residents with dementia living in nursing homes. For residents with dementia living in nursing homes, there is a tension unique to the nursing home environment between ensuring the autonomy of the resident for sexual expression and protecting the resident and other residents from harm. To alleviate this tension, nursing homes will typically conduct an assessment of the resident's capacity for sexual consent. A finding of incapacity should not necessarily preclude the sexual expression of the resident (Syme and Steele, 2016).

Marriage

All capacities are task-specific. Capacity to get married may be the lowest capacity of all (perhaps for good reason) but the specific circumstances in a marriage may require a much higher level of understanding and appreciation — especially in a May—December union with significant impact on different families and property management. (Shulman, 2018)

Financial decisions

A psychiatrist is asked to give an opinion regarding an older adult's ability to manage her finances in a retrospective determination, about a large financial transaction in the past. The older adult has a history of adequate knowledge and skills regarding her financial transactions, but they have declined significantly in recent years. Her current diagnosis of dementia, Alzheimer's type, moderate stage, and cognitive functioning with severely impaired memory, suggests that her memory loss has been present for at least 2—3 years. The examiner's opines that she is not able to make small purchases, write checks, or read or understand her bank statements without assistance.

Financial capacity involves the ability to manage one's financial affairs in a way that is consistent with an older person's personal self-interest and long-standing values. Financial capacity issues often arise in older adults with cognitive impairment. Clinicians are increasingly being asked to give opinions about financial capacity. There are many questions that may be relevant to a clinician's evaluation of financial decision making. Many of these are included in the text box below.

Questions relevant to financial capacity

- What is your financial history? Are you in any debt? Do you live week to week? Are you able to plan ahead and save for the future?
- Do you have enough money to provide for yourself in your retirement?
- Have you made a will?
- How knowledgeable are you about financial investments? What, if any, types of investments do you currently have?
- What are the things you like to spend money on? In spending money, what are your highest priorities?
- Are there people or organizations to who you generally make gifts or contributions? Do I need to use objective capacity measures—what are they?
- How would you like to invest and manage your money in the future? Do you want to stick with what you know, or are you open to new investment options?
- Do you prefer higher-risk investments with a possibility of higher return, or lower-risk investments with a smaller, guaranteed return? Do the choices reflect personal preferences or cultural differences?
- If you needed help with your finances, who would you like to help you? Who can you trust to ensure your best interests?
- How well does this person handle his or her own finances? Is he/she in debt? Does he/she have a good credit record? Is he/she knowledgeable about financial investments?
- Do you currently have or would you like to obtain a financial advisor? Would this person be a more objective spokesperson than a relative or close friend?
- Are there certain people with whom you would like your spokesperson to discuss financial decisions on your behalf (family, financial advisors, other)?
- Is there anyone you specifically would not want to be involved in helping to make financial decisions on your behalf?
- How closely would you want your spokesperson to follow your instructions about financial decisions, versus what he or she thinks is best for you at the time decisions are made?
- Are there other things you would like your spokesperson to know about you, if he or she were ever in a position to make financial decisions on your behalf?

ABA/APA, 2008

Functional elements of financial capacity focus on performance and judgment skills. Financial capacity is complex construct with a range of conceptual and practical skills. The following table, adapted from the clinical

Conceptual model of financial capacity

Basic Monetary Skills	
Naming Coins/Currency	Identify specific coins and currency
Coin/Currency relationships	Indicate monetary values of coins/currency
Counting coins/currency	Accurately count arrays of coins and currency
Financial Conceptual Knowledge	
Define financial concepts	Define simple financial concepts
Apply financial concepts	Practical applications/computation using concepts
Cash Transactions	
Grocery purchase	Conduct 1 item transaction; verify change
Grocery purchase	Conduct 3 item transaction; verify change
Change/vending machine	Obtain change for vending machine; verify charge
Tipping	Understand tipping convention; calculate tips
Checkbook Management	
Understand checkbook	Identify/explain parts of checkbook and register
Use checkbook/register	Conduct simple transaction and pay by check
Bank Statement Management	
Understand bank statement	Identify/explain parts of a bank statement
Use bank statement	Identify specific transactions on bank statement
Financial Judgment	
Detect mail fraud risk	Detect/explain risks in mail fraud solicitation
Detect telephone fraud risk	Detect/explain risks in telephone fraud solicitation
Bill Payment	
Understand bills	Explain meaning and purpose of bills
Prioritize bills	Identify overdue utility bill
Prepare bills for mailing	Prepare bills, checks, envelopes for mailing
Knowledge of Assets/Estate	Indicate personal assets and estate arrangements
Investment Decision Making	Understand investment options; determine returns; make and explain decision
Overall Financial Capacity	**Overall functioning across tasks and domains**

From Ref. ABA/APA 2008 reprinted from Griffith, H.R., Belue, K., Sicola, A., Krzywanski, S., Zamrini, E., Harrell, L., & Marson, D. C. (2003). Impaired financial abilities in mild cognitive impairment: A direct assessment approach. Neurology, 60, 449–457.

model of financial capacity by Marson and colleagues, summarizes some of the key functional elements in financial capacity.

An older person with cognitive impairment may have diminished financial capacity but nevertheless retain preserved financial skills in certain areas. Steps to enhance capacity and accommodations to help an older person needing assistance with financial issues are outlined in the text box below. Caution is advised in this area since older adults with diminished capacity may remain highly vulnerable to financial exploitation despite support. Further text boxes outline additional resources for older adults needing assistance managing their finances, and finally assessment instruments for financial capacity.

Accommodations for the older adult needing help with financial issues

- **Bill paying services** - assist persons with diminished capacity through check depositing, check writing, checkbook balancing, bill paying, insurance claim preparation and filing, tax and public benefit preparation, and counseling
- **Utility company third party notification** - Most utility companies permit customers to designate a third party to be notified by the utility company if bills are not paid on time
- **Shared bank accounts (with family member)** - a common strategy for providing assistance with financial income or assets, it also poses risk in its potential for theft, self-dealing, unintended survivorship, and party account with the family member or friend designated as agent
- **Durable Power of Attorney for finances** - enables a principal to give legal authority, as broadly or as narrowly as desired, to an agent or attorney in fact to act on behalf of the principal, commencing either upon incapacity or commencing immediately and continuing in the event of incapacity. Its creation requires sufficient capacity to understand and establish such an arrangement
- **Trusts** - can be established to serve many purposes, but an important one is the lifetime management of property of one who is or who may become incapacitated. They are especially useful where there is a substantial amount of property at stake and professional management is desired
- **Representative payee** - A person or organization authorized to receive and manage public benefits on behalf of an individual pensions

ABA/APA, 2008

Financial and health-related services available to older persons

- Power of attorney
- Bill paying service
- Joint accounts, joint tenancy

(Continued)

Financial and health-related services available to older persons (*cont'd*)

- Durable power of attorney
- Durable power of attorney for health care
- Representative payee
- Personal trusts
- Limited guardianship
- Plenary guardianship

Holzer et al., 2018

Instruments to assess financial capacity

- Direct Assessment of Functional Status: One subscale
- Decision-making Interview for Guardianship: Four vignettes assessing social judgment in financial situations
- Financial Capacity Instrument: Comprehensive assessment of nine financial domains and overall financial capacity
- Hopemont Capacity Assessment Interview: Three vignettes assessing social judgment in financial situations
- Independent Living Scales: One subscale

ABA/APA, 2008

Testamentary capacity

An 87 year old man has Alzheimer's disease. His attorney drafts a new will in which the man's estate goes to several charities, some of which the attorney either represents or is a significant donor. At the time of the signing, the elderly man could not sign the will or initial the pages, but allegedly made an "x", indicating that he was executing the will.

Finkel, 2008

Testamentary capacity is a legal construct that refers to an individual's ability to make a valid will. Exact definitions of testamentary capacity vary across jurisdictions, but it basically requires three abilities. First, the elder making the will must understand the nature and extent of the property involved (of note, such information need not be exactingly specific, general knowledge is sufficient). Second, the elder must be aware of the natural objects of the property (i.e. immediate or extended family). And third, the elder must know the disposition that such will is making (i.e. who is bequeathed what) (Holzer et al., 2018).

The leading case on testamentary capacity for almost 150 years has been that of Banks versus Goodfellow – a judgment written on appeal by Chief Justice Cockburn of the English High Court in 1870. The broad criteria that emerged from his judgment have formed the basis of virtually every will contest case since that time, despite the fact that a few things have changed since 1870.

Banks versus Goodfellow criteria

In Banks v. Goodfellow (1870), John Banks, the testator (the person executing the will), suffered from a chronic and serious mental illness marked by paranoid delusions and disorganized behavior. However, the court found that none of his delusions affected his ability to understand the relevant facts or the disposition of his assets. The Banks criteria are as follows:

1. Does the testator understand the nature of the will?
2. Does the testator have knowledge of the nature and extent of his assets?
3. Does the testator have knowledge of persons who have a reasonable claim as beneficiaries?
4. Does the testator have an understanding of the impact of distribution of the assets of the estate?
5. Does the testator have any delusions that impact the distribution of assets?
6. Does the testator have the ability to express wishes clearly and consistently?

   Holzer et al., (2018).

Contemporaneous evaluation

Issues to consider prior to contemporaneous assessment of testamentary capacity

Prior to initiating a formal testamentary capacity assessment, there are several factors the potential expert clinician may consider:

- Establish that the expert has adequate medicolegal knowledge and clinical experience to provide an accurate assessment
- Clarify who is requesting the assessment: the testator, the attorney, the family, or an "unnatural" beneficiary
- Discuss retainer and hourly fees as per industry or local practice

(Continued)

Issues to consider prior to contemporaneous assessment of testamentary capacity (*cont'd*)

- Establish who is responsible for the payment of the fees (lawyer or client)
- Clarify expectations regarding the results of a preliminary review, that is, a verbal or written report

Holzer et al., 2018

Upon meeting with the testator, the clinical expert should establish the nature of the relationship, clearly identify the limitations of confidentiality, and explain that information exchanged may be subject to review by the attorneys or the court. The clinical expert should then establish the testator's understanding of the reason for the assessment and possible consequences and obtain informed consent before proceeding.

The clinical interview is the foundation of a contemporaneous evaluation. It is vital that an assessment be conducted in close temporal proximity to the signing of the will. The clinical assessment should include the standard features of a history, mental status, and cognitive exam as well as the specific issues requisite for a finding of testamentary capacity.

The mental status examination would follow the usual format. A detailed probe of thought content is essential given that most American jurisdictions would find testamentary capacity questionable given an "insane delusion". In particular, overvalued ideas, preoccupation, or delusional content in relation to testamentary disposition should be clearly documented. The examiner should assess whether the testator can hold and express views clearly and consistently. Is the testator aware of previous wills? Is the testator aware that a new will revokes a previous will? Is the testator aware of the differences between the previous will and the new will? Is the testator able to provide a rational basis explaining the changes in his or her new will? The clinical expert should maintain detailed records of the testator's understanding of facts and issues, as well as the rationale for any significant changes, especially in a complex or conflictual milieu (Shulman, 2018).

Sensory and language deficits should be screened, and testing to differentiate language functioning from dysphasia may be needed.

In addition to the clinical assessment of the testator, the clinical expert may also find it helpful to review additional material in complex or contested cases: previous wills or codicils, the specific or multiple wills or codicils at issue, a list of the assets corroborated by a collateral source, medical records, psychiatric records, substance abuse treatment records, residential care notes, community care notes, nursing home notes, and assisted living facility notes.

With the testator's consent, the clinician may also interview the spouse, relatives, professional colleagues, personal physicians, and the person drafting the will. Information gained from collateral sources regarding the patient's cognitive functioning would relate to testamentary capacity.

Additional information regarding family conflicts, or paranoid traits, and the testator's attitudes, beliefs, and values could also be helpful (Holzer et al., 2018).

Retrospective evaluation

Recommended steps in conducting a retrospective evaluation of testamentary capacity:

- Identify the operative legal standard for testamentary capacity in your state jurisdiction. For example, in Michigan there are three criteria (Persinger v. Holst, 2001 Michigan Court of Appeals):
  a. To comprehend the nature and extent of his or her property,
  b. To recall the objects of his or her bounty, and
  c. To determine and understand the distribution of his or her property.
- Organize medical, legal, and other records relevant to the capacity issue. Creating a chronological timeline reflecting important medical and lay contacts, and relevant legal transactions, is essential to organizing the information an expert is asked to review.
- Where possible, contact and speak with individuals who knew the decedent testator and can offer informed lay judgments about mental status at the time of will execution.
- Obtain information about the attorneys involved in the will execution. Who was the attorney and what history did he or she have with the adult? Was there a single discussion about the will between the adult and attorney or multiple discussions? Did the attorney make notes at the time the will was created or changed?
- Assess for the presence and severity of a mental disorder at the time of will execution. With older adults, the most often disputed wills are those that were made or modified when an
- individual had a memory disorder or a diagnosed dementia. Is there evidence, through medical records, of a mental disorder that might affect cognitive and emotional abilities related to the elements of testamentary capacity? In some cases, there may be specific neuropsychological test information that will shed light on mental capacity relevant to testamentary capacity.

(Continued)

Recommended steps in conducting a retrospective evaluation of testamentary capacity: (*cont'd*)

- In cases of dementia, seek to determine the stage of dementia as it can significantly inform the clinical judgment of testamentary capacity. The Clinical Dementia Rating (CDR) (Morris, 1993) represents one such dementia staging tool. Because the legal threshold for testamentary capacity is low, an individual with mild dementia may still be capable of making a new will, whereas a patient with more advanced dementia may no longer recognize the objects of his bounty, or know the nature and extent of his property. However, as discussed throughout this handbook, every capacity matter is individual-specific and, irrespective of dementia stage, requires an analysis of the individual's mental status and condition in relation to the particular jurisdictional elements for testamentary capacity.
- Assess testamentary capacity by determining whether there is clinical and other evidence in the record supporting the critical legal elements of this capacity. In some cases, there may be insufficient evidence in the record to support a clinical judgment of testamentary capacity.
- In addition to offering a capacity judgment, a psychologist or other expert is often well-positioned to offer a retrospective opinion regarding the possible role of undue influence in will procurement. Most will contest cases will involve an associated, alternative legal claim of undue influence, with the contention that even if the testator possessed residual testamentary capacity, it was supplanted by the actions of a third-party influencer. Undue influence is discussed in more detail in Chapter 7.

ABA/APA, 2008

Retrospective evaluation refers to the fact that the subject is not available, because he or she is deceased. The evaluation is done posthumously.

Given the principle that capacity is not only task-specific but situation-specific, a simple addition to the criterion may help to provide a more consistent and appropriate approach to this component of the test.

Consider the case of a simple will in an uncomplicated situation where a testator wishes to divide their estate equally between two loving children. Surely, the knowledge of the nature and extent of assets should not be a major concern in the decision about testamentary capacity. On the other hand, a large complicated estate in a conflictual family environment demands a higher threshold of knowledge and appreciation regarding the nature and extent of one's assets and their distribution. If a testator is bequeathing a house to one child and a corporate asset to another, the value of those respective entities is important and must to be tied to the wishes and values of the testator with respect to their beneficiaries. A simple addition to the Banks versus Goodfellow test on this point might be: "Understand the nature and extent of the property relevant to the disposition." This is only one element of Banks versus Goodfellow that could benefit from a refresher after almost 150 years. (Shulman, 2018).

With an increasingly aged, frail population that holds a disproportionate amount of wealth, clinicians (especially those with expertise in older adults) may be asked with more frequency to offer a clinical opinion on testamentary capacity. New decisional instruments are emerging that are designed to assess testamentary capacity contemporaneously, including a semi-structured interview that includes standardized criteria for the legal test for testamentary capacity, supplemented by a validated brief neuropsychological assessment (Brenkel et al., 2018).

Capacity to make end of life decisions

Most Americans living today will cope with one or more chronic conditions for an extended period of time, will spend some years living with disabilities at the end of life (functional and/or cognitive impairment), and will face decisions that may affect the timing and quality of death (Holzer et al., 2018).

Older people do not necessarily fear death — they often fear the loss of their independence and painful illness much more than death itself.

Palliative care, as defined by the World Health Organization, is "an approach that improves the quality of life of patients and their families facing the problems associated with life-threatening illness, through the prevention and relief of suffering by means of early identification and impeccable assessment and treatment of pain and other problems, physical, psychosocial, and spiritual" (Holzer et al., 2018).

Supported and surrogate decision-making

Over time, there has been a transition from transitioned from supported decision-making, where a person with dementia and the caregiver made decisions together, to substituted decision-making, where caregivers took over much decision-making. Points along this continuum represented carers' active involvement in retaining their relative's engagement through providing cues, reducing options, using retrospective information, and using the best interests principle. Practitioners and support services should provide timely advice to caregivers and people with dementia around every day decision-making, and be mindful how abilities may change (Samsi and Manthorpe, 2013). There may be a hierarchy of substitute decision makers, including family members. To help with decision-making, there are various types of services available for older adults. PRACTICAL is a supported decision-making tool for lawyers (American Bar Association Commission on Law and Aging, 2016).

Principles underlying supported and surrogate decision-making

- Substituted judgment is more common, according to which the substitute decision-maker should act as much as possible in accordance with the wish's values and goals of the principle, the different interpretation of those factors in a situation be potentially the basis for conflict
- The best interests approach calls on the agent to perform an objective assessment of the burdens of benefits for this patient as a basis for the decision

ABA/APA, 2008

Guardianship and conservatorship

A 101-year-old woman, who lived alone, broke her hip. On the day she was released from the hospital, her niece and her husband moved in with her. The niece soon had herself named as agent under the older woman's power of attorney, transferred large sums of money to herself and then moved the woman far from her family and friends. The niece changed her phone number, obtained an unlisted number, and turned away visitors who tried to see the woman. The court considered whether to appoint a guardian to replace the niece.

(Frolik, 2001)

Guardianship is judicially determined, based on the presence of persisting impairment of capacity in the absence of a legally designated substitute decision maker. It is among the most common forensic psychiatric evaluations of older adults. Nevertheless, guardianship reports often provide legal decision-makers with inadequate information. Many guardianship evaluations contain conclusory statements about the proposed wards functioning with no description of specific functional impairments (Moye et al., 2007). However, it is no longer enough to assert incapacity and propose guardianship based on a medical diagnosis, as was common in the past. Instead, the standard requires linking decisional impairment to deficits and specific areas of mental functioning.

Ideally, vulnerable individuals will have access to a multiplicity of services and social supports, which optimize functioning and assist with decision-making. Guardianship, as a legal option, should only be used as a last resort when existing supports become inadequate or a legally authorized intervention would bring substantial benefits to the incapable person. Generally, the court seeks to avoid appointing a guardian if less restrictive alternatives exist.

Evaluation for guardianship poses several questions to the clinician forensic evaluator. Important questions for the appointment of a guardian are outlined in the text box below. Clinicians should also bear in mind rapport and the importance of keeping clinical and forensic roles separate. Older people may not have any experience in dealing with government bureaucracy. They may be particularly anxious about formal assessment processes. They may be especially concerned about others trying to force them out of their home and into institutions.

Questions for appointment of a guardian

(1) Does the individual qualify, according to applicable state law, for the appointment of a guardian?

(2) If he or she qualifies, does he or she need a guardian? That is, does the individual have a system of care in place, perhaps an involved relative with durable power of attorney for healthcare finances, that is functioning well? If so, there is no role for the state. Battles over this issue are more commonly seen were power over finances is at stake, but they can also. Guardianship related conflicts (not possible to make a comment here – They can also what? Illogical, and the ending of the sentence doesn't make sense).

(3) The evaluating geriatric psychiatrist may be asked to opine on whether the patient has the capacity to choose his or her guardian, if the court decides that one is needed. That is of course a matter of decisional capacity, not functional capacity per se

Holzer et al., 2018

State guardianship laws: four varying tests of incapacity

- Disabling condition
- Functional behavior (focusing on essential needs)

(Continued)

State guardianship laws: four varying tests of incapacity (*cont'd*)

- Cognitive functioning
- Necessity element or "least restrictive alternative" criteria

APA/APA, 2008

Evaluating guardianship candidates

Despite the considerable interest from psychology and law in how to assess and conceptualize competency issues, relatively little has been written about guardianship, particularly how to best evaluate guardianship candidates. This is problematic because a guardian is assigned once an individual is adjudicated incompetent and decision-making about this is difficult in some cases.

Mental health professionals have much to offer the court in making recommendations about a suitable guardian. Domains that should be assessed include the following: relationship with proposed ward, knowledge and insight about proposed ward, guardianship plans, decision-making style, and suitability for guardianship. Recommendations are also provided for especially difficult cases such as when working with families in conflict, the presence of undue influence, and when a family member or friend is pitted against a disinterested public agency (Demakis, 2016).

10 tips for thorough evaluations for guardianship

1. Consider the context of the consultation. This includes medical factors (such as the patient's condition, prognosis, relationship with the treatment team, and recommended course of treatment), legal factors (e.g. pending litigation and relevant legal standards for issues such as guardianship), and psychosocial issues (e.g. the patient's current support structure and family conflicts)
2. Identify the legal issue and any relevant legal standards. The legal standard will inform you of the issues you need to address in the evaluation. If an attorney has consulted you, ask him or her to provide the legal standard
3. Gather relevant collateral information, which may include interviews with family members or a review of financial or medical records
4. Explain the purpose of the examination and the limits of confidentiality

10 tips for thorough evaluations for guardianship (*cont'd*)

5. Perform a focused psychiatric evaluation, paying special attention to cognitive functioning, reasoning, and unusual thought content such as delusional beliefs
6. Perform an interview specific to the referral issue
7. Consider using a relevant assessment instrument
8. Consider psychological testing, laboratory testing, imaging, or further medical evaluation. These assessments can help determine the diagnosis, the cause of any deficits in capacity, and whether any deficits are reversible
9. Determine what opinions you are able to render. Limit opinions and remember that it may be appropriate to decline to address certain issues if there is insufficient information or if the issue is outside your area of expertise
10. Prepare a written report. Consider the audience. Minimize the use of medical jargon and define all medical terms. State your opinions clearly and with reasonable medical certainty (in most jurisdictions, this means more likely than not). State the basis for all opinions

Soliman, 2012

Guardianship reform

A groundbreaking 1987 Associated Press (AP) series triggered modern guardianship reform, contending that "overworked and understaffed court systems frequently break down, abandoning those incapables of caring for themselves" (Bayles & McCartney, Guardians of the Elderly: An Ailing System, 1987).

Challenges to guardianship reform

Making lasting change in guardianship is challenging because:

1. Practices differ significantly by state and by court
2. Cases are complex—often fraught with issues of mental illness, medication, family discord, undue influence, abuse and exploitation, service provider fragmentation, and lack of resources
3. Guardians constantly walk a fine line negotiating risks, protections, and self-determination, often with little guidance
4. Resources are limited—funds, data, and research are scarce

https://www.americanbar.org/groups/law_aging/resources/wings-court-stakeholder-partnerships0/guardianship-reform-wings-background/.

Conclusion

The geriatric forensic evaluator who applies a comprehensive approach for capacity and guardianship questions takes time to get to know the evaluee as a person, and ensures that the evaluee has been adequately informed. He or she helps to ensure that older adults live their lives in a way that is consistent with their values and goals.

Selected references

ABA/APA Assessment of Capacity in Older Adults Project Working Group, American Bar Association Commission on Law and Aging, American Psychological Association, 2008. Assessment of Older Adults with Diminished Capacity: A Handbook for Psychologists. American Bar Association Commission on Law and Aging: American Psychological Association, Washington, D.C.

American Bar Association Commission on Law and Aging, C.o.D.R., Section on Civil Rights and Social Justice; and Section on Real Property, Trust and Estate Law, 2016. Practical Tool for Lawyers: Steps in Supporting Decision-Making.

American Geriatrics Society, 2016. Clinician's Guide to Assessing and Counseling Older Drivers, third ed. New York. Available at: https://www.nhtsa.gov/sites/nhtsa.dot.gov/files/812228_cliniciansguidetoolderdrivers.pdf.

Appelbaum, P.S., 1998. Ought we to require emotional capacity as part of decisional competence? Kennedy Inst. Ethics J. 8 (4), 377–387.

Appelbaum, P.S., Grisso, T., 1988. Assessing patients' capacities to consent to treatment. N. Engl. J. Med. 319 (25), 1635–1638.

Appelbaum, P.S., Bonnie, R.J., Karlawish, J.H., 2005. The capacity to vote of persons with Alzheimer's disease. Am. J. Psychiatry 162 (11), 2094–2100.

Brenkel, M., Whaley, K., Herrmann, N., Crawford, K., Hazan, E., Cardiff, L., Owen, A.M., Shulman, K., 2018. A case for the standardized assessment of testamentary capacity. Can. Geriatr. J. 21 (1), 26–31.

Buchanan, A., 2004. Mental capacity, legal competence and consent to treatment. J. R. Soc. Med. 97 (9), 415–420.

Bush, S., Allen, R., Heck, A., Moye, J., 2015. Ethical issues in geropsychology: clinical and forensic perspectives. Psychol. Injury Law 8 (4), 348–356.

Chen, S.T., Sultzer, D.L., Hinkin, C.H., Mahler, M.E., Cummings, J.L., 1998. Executive dysfunction in Alzheimer's disease: association with neuropsychiatric symptoms and functional impairment. J. Neuropsychiatry Clin. Neurosci. 10 (4), 426–432.

Demakis, G.J., 2016. Evaluating potential guardians for adults adjudicated incompetent. Arch. Clin. Neuropsychol. 31 (6), 562–569.

Di Napoli, E.A., Breland, G.L., Allen, R.S., 2013. Staff knowledge and perceptions of sexuality and dementia of older adults in nursing homes. J. Aging Health 25 (7), 1087–1105.

Dunn, L.B., Fisher, S.R., Hantke, M., Appelbaum, P.S., Dohan, D., Young, J.P., Roberts, L.W., 2013. Thinking about it for somebody else: Alzheimer's disease research and proxy decision makers' translation of ethical principles into practice. Am. J. Geriatr. Psychiatry 21 (4), 337–345.

Finkel, S., 2008. The role of the geriatric specialist in regards to the marginal testator. Trusts Estates 32. https://www.wealthmanagement.com/data-amp-tools/april-2008.

Frolik, L.A., 2001. The strange interplay of testamentary capacity and the doctrine of undue influence. Are we protecting older testators or overriding individual preferences? Int. J. Law Psychiatry 24 (2–3), 253–266.

Ganzini, L., Volicer, L., Nelson, W.A., Fox, E., Derse, A.R., 2004. Ten myths about decision-making capacity. J. Am. Med. Dir. Assoc. 5 (4), 263–267.
Gold, L.H., Vanderpool, D.L., 2013. Clinical Guide to Mental Disability Evaluations, xxv. Springer, New York, p. 394.
Grisso, T., Applebaum, P.S., 1998. Assessing Competence to Consent to Treatment: A Guide for Physicians and Other Health Professionals. Oxford University Press, New York.
Grosso, T., 1986. Evaluating competencies, NY: Plenum.
Holzer, J.C., Kohn, R., Ellison, J.M., Recupero, P.R., 2018. Geriatric Forensic Psychiatry: Principles and Practice. Oxford University Press, New York, NY.
Lai, J.M., Karlawish, J., 2007. Assessing the capacity to make everyday decisions: a guide for clinicians and an agenda for future research. Am. J. Geriatr. Psychiat. 15 (2), 101–111.
Morris, C.J., Nov 1993. The Clinical Dementia Rating (CDR). Neurology 43 (11), 2412–2412-a. https://doi.org/10.1212/WNL.43.11.2412-a.
Moye, J., Sabatino, C.P., Brendel, R.W., 2013a. Evaluation of the capacity to appoint a healthcare proxy. Am. J. Geriatr. Psychiatry 21 (4), 326–336.
Moye, J., Marson, D.C., Edelstein, B., 2013b. Assessment of capacity in an aging society. Am. Psychol. 68 (3), 158.
Moye, J., Wood, S., Edelstein, B., Armesto, J.C., Bower, E.H., Harrison, J.A., Wood, E., 2007. Clinical evidence in guardianship of older adults is inadequate: findings from a tri-state study. Gerontologist 47 (5), 604–612.
Ontario (2010) Government Capacity Assessor Resources.
O'Reilly, R.L., 2008. The capacity to execute an advance directive for psychiatric treatment. Int. J. Law Psychiatry 31 (1), 66–71.
Overton, E., Appelbaum, P.S., Fisher, S.R., Dohan, D., Roberts, L.W., Dunn, L.B., 2013. Alternative decision-makers' perspectives on assent and dissent for dementia research. Am. J. Geriatr. Psychiatry 21 (4), 346–354.
Pomidor, A. (Ed.), 2019. Clinician's Guide to Assessing and Counseling Older Drivers, 4th Edition. The American Geriatrics Society, New York.
Roth, L.H., Meisel, A., Lidz, C.W., 1977. Tests of competency to consent to treatment. Am. J. Psychiatry 134 (3), 279–284.
Samsi, K., Manthorpe, J., 2013. Everyday decision-making in dementia: findings from a longitudinal interview study of people with dementia and family carers. Int. Psychogeriatr. 25 (6), 949–961.
Shulman, K., 2018. All about Estates – Blog Posts 2014–2016 from. https://www.allaboutestates.ca/author/kshulman/.
Simpson, J.R., 2014. DSM-5 and neurocognitive disorders. J. Am. Acad. Psychiat. Law 42 (2), 159–164.
Society, A.G., 2016. Clinician's Guide to Assessing and Counseling Older Drivers, third ed. New York.
Soliman, S., 2012. Evaluating older adults' capacity and need for guardianship: 10 steps to ensure your assessments are thorough, accurate, and fair. Curr. Psychiat. 11 (4), 39–54.
Syme, M.L., Steele, D., 2016. Sexual consent capacity assessment with older adults. Arch. Clin. Neuropsychol. 31 (6), 495–505.
Wilkins, J. (2016) "Ethical considerations regarding capacity assessments for consent to sexual activity in older adults with dementia living in residential care settings." Am. J. Geriatr. Psychiat. 23(3): S113.

CHAPTER FIVE

Evaluation of elder abuse and financial exploitation

Contents

Elder abuse

Elder abuse is a growing societal concern, affecting at least 1 in 10 older Americans. Researchers and practitioners alike consistently assert that a dramatic discrepancy exists between the actual rates of elder abuse versus the number of elder abuse cases reported. As a field of study, the recognition and understanding of elder abuse are still emerging. Comparing findings of a small, but growing, body of literature that cover perceived and substantiated cases of elder abuse is challenging because there is no uniform term or agreed-upon definition, used among state governments, researchers, health care and service providers, and advocates (Roberto, 2016).

Elder abuse is often a silent issue in clinical settings. However, it is a global concern, affecting millions of older people worldwide, and a focus on increasing international concern. Elder abuse is a pervasive and growing problem, urgently requiring the attention of geriatric psychiatrists, hospitals,

The Clinician's Guide to Geriatric Forensic Evaluations
ISBN: 978-0-12-815034-4
https://doi.org/10.1016/B978-0-12-815034-4.00005-2

health care systems, social services, lawmakers and communities. Elder abuse is a problem that is larger than previously thought and without geographic boundaries. It is a prevalent, identifiable and costly problem with the increasing number of aging adults in the world.

Clinicians working with older adults have all had patients who are victims of elder abuse, though we may not be aware of it. Many older adults are ashamed of their experiences and hide the facts of their abuse from physicians and mental health professionals. Clinicians should keep in mind the possibility of abuse, even if a vulnerable patient denies it. Perpetrators of elder abuse are often someone the elder knows and trusts.

Mistreated older adults tend to deny that abuse or neglect is taking place, or refuse to report it, which results in underreporting. Determination of the prevalence of elder abuse is biased—not only because of underreporting but also due to difficulties obtaining data from cognitively impaired people, those with hearing loss and/or those who are physically frail. Privacy is another factor discouraging some elders from speaking up about abuse.

Older victims of abuse may not report abuse because of: [1] fear of retaliation, [2] being removed from the home, [3] because they believe that the abuse was deserved, [4] a belief that there is nowhere else to go, [5] a belief that nothing can be done about it or [6] shame surrounding such treatment from one's own family (Kosberg and Garcia, 1995).The elder may also be concerned that family members may face criminal charges. Furthermore, elderly victims may be fearful that removing the abuser removes physical support, care and/or financial support which is standing between elder and long-term care.

Two national studies on the prevalence of elder abuse have been conducted in the United States. The first study found rates of 9.0% for verbal abuse, 0.2% for physical abuse and 3.5% for financial mistreatment. The second study, which was a larger use random digit dialing, found a one-year prevalence of 4.6% for emotional abuse, 1.6% for physical abuse, 0.6% for sexual abuse, 5.1% for potential neglect and 5.2% for financial abuse. One in 10 elders had experienced some form of abuse in the past year (Acierno et al., 2010). The incidence of elder abuse is many times, one study estimated 24 times, greater than the number of cases referred to social service, law enforcement, and other legal authorities. Victims of elder abuse are three times more likely to die in a three-year period. The few studies that have examined the prevalence of elder abuse in nursing facilities have suggested it is not an uncommon occurrence.

Risk factors for elder abuse

Both patient and caregiver factors are associated with elder abuse. While women are more likely to be victims of sexual and physical assault, men are more likely to die from homicide due to neglect (Shields, 2004). Caregiver factors, rather than risk factors associated with the abused elder, may be more important in predicting abuse and neglect (Reis, 1998). For example, anxious and depressed caregivers engage in more abuse than other caregivers of individuals with dementia (Cooper, 2010).

Victim and caregiver risk factors for elder physical & emotional abuse, and neglect:

- Victim factors
- Older
- Lower socioeconomic status
- Cognitive impairment
- Mental illness
- Substance use disorder
- Assistance with activities of daily living
- Physical dependence
- Emotional dependence
- Financial dependence
- Poor social support
- Submissive
- Withdrawal
- Demanding
- Aggressive
- Provocative
- Previously blue abused
- Poor communication

Holzer et al., 2018, p. 174

Caregiver factors

- Responsible for elder greater than age 75
- Male
- Children greater than spouse
- Mental illness
- Substance use disorder
- I met activity of daily living needs
- Poor physical health
- Dependent on the elder

(Continued)

Caregiver factors (*cont'd*)

- Social isolation
- Poor social supports
- Stressed
- Aggressive, hostile
- Relationship conflict
- Living with dependent elder
- Unwilling caregiver
- High expectations of elder

Few data sets exist regarding the characteristics of professional caregivers who abuse residents in nursing home facilities, however the following risk factors for employees who become abusive have been identified:

Caregiver risk factors for elder abuse in nursing home settings

- Lower job satisfaction
- Viewing patients as childlike
- Experiencing burnout
- Loss of immunity (ability for staff to resist responding to abuse from aggressive nursing home residents)
- Due to difficult work environments
- History of domestic violence
- History of mental illness,
- Drug or alcohol dependence

Council 2003

Mental health consequences of elder abuse

- Fear
- Psychological distress
- Anxiety
- Depression
- Post-traumatic stress disorder

Dong 2017

Common physical findings in elder abuse

- Bruises
- Burns
- Rashes

Common physical findings in elder abuse (*cont'd*)

- Ulcers
- Head injuries
- Strangulation marks
- Fractures

Confronting and reducing elder abuse require a multisectoral and multidisciplinary approach. Historically, elder abuse was approached with a social services response, but with the passing in 2017 of the Elder Abuse Prevention and Prosecution Act, criminalization of elder abuse is the new direction.

Definition

What is elder abuse? Elder abuse is a broad term. No single definition describes elder abuse uniformly across legal jurisdictions, or across various countries, states, medical subspecialties, organizations, and research studies.

Definitions of elder abuse

- A generally accepted definition of elder abuse is one proposed by the US National Academy of Sciences: accidents that cause harm, whether or not harm as intended, to a vulnerable elder by a caregiver or other person who stands in a trust relationship to the elder or failure by caregiver to satisfy the elders basic needs or to protect elder from harm.
- *The Elder Justice Roadmap Report* uses the following definition of elder abuse: physical, sexual or psychological abuse, as well as neglect, and/or financial exploitation of an older person by another person or entity, that occurs in any setting, such as a home, community, or a facility, in a relationship where there is an expectation of trust and/or when an older person is targeted based on age or disability (Connolly, 2014).
- The Centers for Disease Control and Prevention (CDC) developed uniform definitions for elder abuse (CDC, 2018) elder abuse surveillance uniform definitions and recommendations. An intentional act or failure to act by a caregiver or another person in a relationship involving the expectation of trust that causes or creates a risk of harm to an older adult.

In all of the above definitions of elder abuse, the abusive act is committed by a caregiver or person in a position of trust or in an institutional setting, which defines elder abuse or other crimes, violence and/or exploitation of an elderly individual.

Common elements in formal definitions of elder abuse include:

- An act of commission or omission
- May be intentional or unintentional abuse or neglect
- Can be perpetrated by the victim, a trusted other, a stranger, or an acquaintance
- Can occur in domestic or institutional settings
- Results in harm or threatened harm to the health or welfare of an older adult
- Harm can be physical, psychological, social, financial, or sexual

Overall, the legal definition of elder abuse differs considerably from state to state in the United States. The types of abuse that fall under the law and the definition of abuse also vary. Some states include acts committed by non-caregivers or institutions of care to be elder abuse. Other states narrow the definition to only vulnerable adults. The definition of who qualifies as an elder varies by age or may be undefined. As the American indigenous populations are sovereign, they are governed by different sets of laws.

Types of elder abuse

Elder mistreatment has been examined from a broad perspective to include collective or societal abuse, institutional abuse, and individual abuse. Collective abuse of older people includes ageism and discrimination, in areas such as the right to autonomy, healthcare decision-making, education, and employment. Institutional elder abuse includes refusal of care, regulatory violations, Medicare and other financial fraud, as well as other criminal actions by health- care organizations. The term elder abuse, however, is typically limited to individual abuse. Although self-neglect, where the elder refuses care, has at times been folded into the broader concept of elder abuse, it is not considered to be elder abuse from a geriatric forensic psychiatry perspective. There are five principal domains of elder abuse: [1] physical abuse, [2] emotional or psychological abuse, both verbal and nonverbal, [3] sexual abuse, [4] neglect and [5] financial abuse.

Allegations of elder abuse and neglect

An 80 year old man with Lewy body dementia experiences deterioration in his condition, leaving him unable to speak during his final months. As his health worsened, his wife prevented any contact with her husband, particularly by his children by his first marriage. The children later protested in front of his home, having not been allowed contact with their father for months. Longtime friends and colleagues

Allegations of elder abuse and neglect (*cont'd*)

also joined the demonstration. The older children sought conservatorship over their father's care; the court denied their petition. The man was removed from a nursing home by his wife. A judge ordered separate visitation times for the man's wife and his children from his first marriage.

The CDC has also provided the following definitions of each form of abuse: [1] physical abuse, [2] sexual abuse, [3] emotional or psychological abuse, [4] neglect, and [5] financial abuse or exploitation.

Types of elder abuse:

- Physical Abuse
- Sexual Abuse
- Emotional Abuse
- Neglect
- Financial Exploitation
- Self-Neglect

Physical abuse refers to the use of force resulting in injury, pain, or impairment. Threats of harm may be part of physical abuse. Injuries due to neglect may also be due to abuse by a caregiver, such as bone fractures, inadequate medical care, malnutrition/cachexia, or decubitus ulcers.

Emotional (psychological) abuse results in anguish, pain or other distress, due to verbal (insults, harassment, humiliation) or non-verbal acts. It is often associated with physical abuse. Emotional abuse may be part of efforts to manipulate or isolate the elder.

Financial abuse (elder financial exploitation) is common and may involve the disposition of a person's estate, gifts, property transfers, and other financial acts. It may be more likely to be identified by the victim's family or financial professionals than by physicians.

Sexual abuse refers to non-consensual sexual contact. It includes not only rape but other types of sexual assault, including unwanted exposure to nudity. Elders are vulnerable to sexual abuse since they are often cared for in settings where there is little supervision of the caregiver, who may be a stranger.

Neglect is mistreatment resulting from inadequate attention, carelessness or disregard for an individual's needs. It can encompass physical, emotional, abandonment, financial and self-neglect issues.

Elder mistreatment and undue influence

An elderly widow and philanthropist served on the boards of many cultural institutions. Her only son was found guilty of criminal charges after swindling millions from his mother after she was stricken with Alzheimer's disease. In the criminal trial, prosecution witnesses portrayed a confused, disoriented and sometimes paranoid woman, who forgot the names of longtime friends, mistook her son for her long-deceased husband and could not have been lucid when she made her son the sole executor of of her sizeable estate. Prosecutors said the son had been driven to inflate his inheritance at the urging of his wife.

Elder abuse situations rarely come to the attention of authorities. The scope of elder abuse has been a subject of interest and speculation for decades. Very few studies have used professional surveys or official data to examine the incidence, prevalence, or mortality of elder abuse. Some studies suggest there may be patterns of verbal mistreatment for women and those with physical disabilities being more common. Financial abuse is usually more prevalent for those without a spouse or intimate partner. Interventions that have the potential to prevent mistreatment include caregiver interventions, money management programs, helplines, emergency shelters, and multidisciplinary teams.

He wouldn't turn me loose

96-year-old Miss Mary was financially exploited and later, sexually assaulted by her grandson. Miss Mary had been living with her grandson and his wife for five years during which financial abuse took place. Then, one evening, when his wife was out, the grandson sexually abused Miss Mary for several hours, leaving her bruised from head to toe.

After the attack and hospitalization, Miss Mary was placed in a nursing home under the name "Jane Doe" for safety reasons. Miss Mary's family refused to believe her and refused to support her; her primary social interactions were with staff and residents of the nursing home, and the advocates she met after the assault. However, Miss Mary retained her strength of character, and fully participated in the subsequent trial and prosecution of her grandson.

Source: Terra Nova Films (2012)

Clinical evaluation of elder abuse

Concerns about elder abuse may arise at home, in nursing homes or other residential settings. Elements of abuse may become evident in the course of the clinical evaluation. There may have been recent changes or decline in functioning which would gain the clinician's attention.

The evaluation of elder abuse begins with an initial psychiatric assessment that should be standard for all geriatric patients seen by a mental health professional. A thorough social history is necessary to capture exposure to trauma, the quality of relationships, in particular, those with those residing in their own household and their knowledge of their finances (Lichtenberg, 2016). As individuals with dementia are at high risk for abuse, careful cognitive assessments and evaluation of independence and activities of daily living and instrumental activities of daily living are necessary. The psychiatric assessment may re-raise red flags of suspected elder abuse and may necessitate reporting to adult protective services.

Depending on state regulations, interviewing caregivers and the alleged perpetrator may provide further useful information. Perpetrators will rarely acknowledge elder abuse. If an abused elder has a mental illness this should be treated. A safety plan should be drawn up and interventions provided based on the situation. Neglect, financial, verbal, physical or sexual abuse each may require different specific interventions. If the abused individual has a major cognitive or neurocognitive disorder, a determination of their decision-making capacity to refuse or accept interventions may be necessary.

Older people may not have much experience in dealing with government bureaucracy. They may be particularly anxious about formal assessment processes. They may resent any government involvement in their affairs.

Multiple screening instruments are available to assess elder abuse, but none are in widespread use in geriatric psychiatry settings. Medical and psychiatric care is fundamental in the identification and management of such situations. The first step in evaluation is to conduct a comprehensive geriatric psychiatric assessment, including a mental status examination with screening for mood and psychotic disorders. The degree of cognitive impairment may be assessed using a standard brief rating scale such as the Montreal Cognitive Assessment (MoCA), the Mini-Mental State Examination (MMSE), or a clock-drawing test. The executive function should be evaluated since this is the major cognitive domain associated with decision-making. Moreover, collateral information should be obtained from caregivers and concerned parties, while maintaining an open mind to the possibility of abuse, even with established patients and familiar caregivers. The psychiatrist may need additional knowledge of key facts from outside sources to reliably assess an older person's memory.

Careful physical examination is recommended, paying special attention to possible injuries, bearing in mind that many older people are prone to falls or bedsores and that they may have fractures or other injuries for reasons other than abuse. Geriatric psychiatrists suspecting elder abuse should arrange for the victim to be physically examined by an appropriate specialist. Clinicians should be alert to any inappropriate use of drugs, restraints or punishment.

Interviewing techniques for elder abuse

The clinical interview provides an opportunity to the geriatric psychiatrist to gain greater knowledge of the victim's situation. However, it may not be helpful to directly question an older adult about abuse. Some patients may be ashamed and reluctant to admit they have been abused, while other abused elders may not conceive of themselves as victims, believing they are dependent and need the abuser to take care of their affairs.

Language and cultural barriers can be a major obstacle to identifying elder abuse. Elders from ethnic, sexual or religious minorities may be particularly vulnerable. They may need to be interviewed using a translator or other mediator. Family members, especially the patient's children, should not be used as translators, since these individuals may themselves be the perpetrators. Moreover, using an elder's children as translators can convey disrespect. Professional translators or a phone translation service should be used whenever possible since it's important to obtain objective and verifiable information.

Clinical tips: legal and ethical issues in elder abuse cases

In cases of elder abuse and suspected elder abuse, there are complex ethical and legal issues that must be considered: [1] Avoid role conflicts and dual role relationships where possible. Consider referring the patient for an independent forensic opinion rather than mixing up the responsibilities of clinical and forensic roles. [2] Be mindful of patient confidentiality if called to court in response to a subpoena. [3] Have procedures in place that clarify the relationship, fees, and expectations for your forensic work. [4] Obtain specific legal decision-making capacity for different tasks including the capacity to manage finances, sign a contract, marry or make a will [5] Informed consent may be difficult to obtain from an older person in cases of diminished capacity. [6] Clinicians should consider seeking professional legal advice from attorneys or from their malpractice carrier if questions arise about how to manage legal and ethical aspects of elder abuse situations.

Documentation and reporting

Thorough documentation is very important in elder abuse situations. The medical record may later comprise critical evidence in legal proceedings about the documented abuse. Clinicians should record their observations carefully and thoroughly, including mental status examination findings, cognitive findings, quotations from the older victim, photographs (in the case of physical abuse findings) and always clarifying sources of collateral information.

Jurisdictions vary widely in their requirements to report elder abuse. Reporting is often done on a confidential basis. Clinicians should learn the requirements that are applicable in are where they work. Nursing homes and other institutions may have special reporting requirements and procedures.

Adult protective services

The term protective services encompass a broad range of services. It includes various social services voluntarily received by seniors in need of support (e.g., homemaker or chore services, nutrition programs). It also includes interventions for persons who may be abused, neglected, or exploited, and which may lead to some form of guardianship.

Elder financial exploitation

Elder financial exploitation or victimization is defined by the U.S. Administration on Aging as the "illegal or improper use of the financial or material resources of an older individual for monetary or personal benefit, profit or gain." This definition is not limited to caregivers. Elder financial victimization can be classified into four broad categories: [1] door-to-door scams, [2] professional swindles, and [3] abuse by professionals in a position of trust, such as bankers, financial advisors, attorneys, religious leaders, doctors, caregivers, friends, and acquaintances.

According to a 2011 MetLife study (The MetLife Study, 2011), which used data from the Administration on Aging's National Center on Elder Abuse, an estimated $ 2.9 billion is lost annually by victims of elder financial victimization. Financial abuse often occurs simultaneously with other forms of abuse, such as 12.1% caregiver neglect, 5.1% physical abuse, and 3.8% psychological abuse. Career criminals who deliberately prey on the elderly establish control over them and then use deceit and intimidation to steal from them.

Types of scams targeting elders

- Door-to-door scam: usually a one-time occurrence, an individual comes to elder's door and falsely represents themselves as a repairman, skilled worker, or charity representative, contracting for services he or she does not provide, double-billing for services, or collecting money under the guise of charity.
- Professional swindle: a more elaborate scheme that evolves over months or years and can involve large amounts of money.
- "Nigerian prince scam: a swindler sends an email asking for a loan or monetary advance with the promise that there will be a large return on the elder's investment, which, of course, never materializes
- "Grandparent scam: a scammer randomly dials an elder and then poses as a grandchild, convincing the grandparent to wire money for an urgent expense, such as bail from a foreign jail or a dire medical bill. The scammer intentionally pressures the elder into sending money immediately, in order to leave no time to debunk the story by checking with family members.
- Domestic financial abuse: though not the most common type of financial victimization reported to authorities, is likely vastly underreported and is estimated to account for approximately 90% of financial abuse

Holzer et al., 2018

One useful model for conceptualizing how financial abuse occurs is IDEAL Model (ABA/APA, 2008).

IDEAL model for elder financial exploitation and undue influence (Blum, in APA/ABA, 2008)

- Isolation from social contacts
- Dependency on the perpetrator
- Emotional manipulation or exploitation of vulnerability
- Acquiescence to the perpetrator
- Loss financially

Manipulation or exploitation of the victim can occur through fraud, in which the perpetrator confuses the victim or keeps him or her unaware of the financial transactions that are taking place. This can also occur through coercion, in which the perpetrator uses intimidation and threats to persuade the victim to go along with the financial transactions (Wilber and Reynolds, 1997). Often there is methodical isolation of victims from friends and relatives to leave them more vulnerable to subsequent abuse.

The greatest risk factor for financial victimization is age. Individuals over age 80 are at highest risk. One simple reason is that older individuals are most commonly targeted because of their financial reserves. Individuals over age 50 control more than 70% of the country's wealth and household headed by individuals aged 75 and older have the highest median net worth of any age group. Data from 1996 showed that 40% of the population over the age of 70 had a net worth ranging from $171,000-$485,000.

Other risk factors for financial victimization include being female, a lack of familiarity with managing finances (i.e. a recently deceased spouse who always handled the finances), physical or emotional health, social isolation, debridement and/or cognitive impairment. A study found the victims of substantial financial abuse had overall poor memory, lower calculation speeds, slower speech processing, and below average executive functioning. These neuropsychological domains are key to appropriately managing finances, and they may be the first to go in the course of neurodegenerative illness. Therefore, financial management capacity can be seriously compromised before other decisional capacities are affected (Wood, 2014).

Perpetrators, usually family members, frequently have low self-esteem, significant psychosocial stress, caregiver burden, and possible substance abuse.

Financial victimization can be devastating to the elder, leading to depression, hopelessness, suicide, social withdrawal and even repeat victimization. Victims are four times more likely than non-victims to be admitted to nursing homes and three times more likely to be admitted to the hospital. Frequently, there is reluctance from victims to report financial abuse. Barriers to reporting include guilt and shame, fear of retaliation from the perpetrator, fear of abandonment and fear of having to move into a nursing home. Fear of abandonment is the most pronounced for those physically dependent on the perpetrator as a primary caregiver. The lack of a standardized national reporting mechanism for financial abuse makes it even more difficult for victims to speak up, and many fear having to involve the police and what that process will entail. Even when reported, cases of financial abuse are rarely prosecuted (Navarro et al., 2013).

Financial exploitation: suspicious caregiver behaviors

- Caregiver shows excessive interest in elders finances
- Caregiver does not allow Elder to speak for him or herself and insist on being present, assign Also seen in other forms of elder abuse
- New best friends are sweethearts in the elder's life
- Caregiver suddenly acquires expensive new possessions
- Elder acts withdrawn, submissive, or feel for fearful toward the caregiver

Clinical screening for financial victimization requires overcoming a natural reluctance to ask patients about private financial matters. Patients should be interviewed alone and asked about their finances, recent transactions, necessary documentation, the quality of family relationships, caregivers, and friends. Their capacity to make financial decisions should also be assessed.

Red flags for financial abuse, finances and interactions with caregiver

- Finances
- Unpaid bills or eviction notices
- Unusual bank account activity
- Attempts to wire large amounts of money
- Bank statements no longer coming to home
- Beneficiary changes in will or insurance policy
- Suspicious signatures on checks and documents
- Elder is reluctant or unable to discuss financial matters

Holzer et al., 2018

Undue influence

Susceptible to undue influence?

Mr. J, eighty-eight years old and a widower, approached his longtime attorney to make changes in his estate planning and will. At that time, his grandson was living in Mr. J's home, assisting with some of his care, and attending college. Mr. J had four adult children and six grandchildren. A previous will had split his estate equally

Susceptible to undue influence? (*cont'd*)

among his children, with no specific mention of grandchildren. Now he wanted to change his will to leave his current home to his grandson, and to provide funds to pay for his grandson's tuition. The estate attorney requested an evaluation of capacity and susceptibility to undue influence based upon the client's age, and the increased possibility of litigation given the shift from past dispositions.

Wood and Liu 2012

Undue influence refers to the substitution of a person's wishes or free will with someone else's wishes. It is a legal construct, defined by the courts. The approach to undue influence varies in different jurisdictions. Geriatric forensic evaluators may be asked to give an opinion about undue influence after assessing impairments and factors making an older individual vulnerable.

Questions about undue influence can arise in a variety of medical or legal contexts: primarily wills, but also contracts including power of attorney. Expert evaluation for undue influence is frequently performed retrospectively after the testator, or person making the will, is deceased.

Undue influence is a complex concept. At a basic level, it involves the substitution of a person's wishes with the wishes of the influencer. It is distinguished from "due" influence (natural favoritism or devotion to certain heirs) in that undue influence involves coercion (often over an extended period of time, and it may be concealed or indirect) and personal control over the testator. There is rarely direct evidence of undue influence, so courts generally make this determination based on circumstantial evidence, by relying on inference. Undue influence is a distinct concept from fraud (e.g. deception, trickery, forgery) and duress (e.g. direct threats of harm, blackmail).

Unlike testamentary capacity, which has relatively well defined and widely accepted criteria (Banks vs. Goodfellow), there is no clear consensus on the precise definition of undue influence. Several sets of criteria have been developed to define and conceptualize undue influence, but none is in universal use.

There may be allegations that the patient is subject to undue influence, having made decisions that reflect the influence of another with ulterior motives. The availability of informants may be helpful in the evaluation process, as well as important sources of collateral information. A competing issue, however, may involve the context of the evaluation and whether other informants have secondary involvement or gain, such as family or significant others' involvement.

Evaluations to examine the potential presence of undue influence require knowledge of several concepts:

- **Capacity:** Broadly refers to an individual's ability to receive and evaluate information and make and express a decision.
- **Financial Exploitation:** A type of elder abuse, involving the improper use or theft of another's assets.
- **Undue Influence:** When exploiters, whether family, acquaintances, or strangers, use their power to *deceptively* gain control over the decision making of a victim. Often involves financial exploitation.

ABA/APA (2008, p.113)

Perpetrator Tactics for elder financial exploitation

- Isolate from others and information
- Create fear
- Prey on vulnerabilities
- Create dependency
- Create lack of faith in own abilities
- Induce shame and secrecy
- Perform intermittent acts of kindness
- Keep victim unaware

ABA/APA Psychologist's Guide, p. 116

Reliable instruments are not available to measure susceptibility to undue influence and coercion. Unfortunately, this results in a wide spectrum of accepted and common medical and legal practices, which may yield widely varying outcomes, which are often to the detriment of the patient and their family. It can be difficult to probe insight, awareness, concern, organization, planning or the understanding of consequences (Shulman et al., 2007).

Her friend, the contractor

Ms. K, a seventy-seven-year-old woman, developed a relationship with a contractor after she discovered they shared a passion for aviation. The contractor had been living in a garage apartment while completing work on the main home. After about two months, he moved into the main home and developed a close friendship with

Her friend, the contractor (*cont'd*)

Ms. K. She gave him permission to use her private plane housed at a nearby airport. Neighbors reported that Ms. K had been less social and reluctant to talk about her new friend. They indicated that she had also demonstrated changes in her habits, which included purchasing new furnishings and a car when she had been noted to be very frugal in times past. Ms. K was divorced and had no children. Her sister was still living, and their relationship was civil but not close. After about six months, Ms. K fell and was hospitalized for a broken hip. Her friend, the contractor, visited her at the hospital with some legal documents, including a power of attorney and a quitclaim deed. Following her hospitalization, he had her moved to an assisted living facility on the far side of the community; he moved into her main home and continued to use her plane. After her death a few months later, her revised estate plans came to light, leaving everything to the new friend. Her sister contested the new will, raising concerns of undue influence.

Wood 2012

Weapons of influence

In his 1984 book *Influence: The Psychology of Persuasion*, based on three undercover years applying for and training at used car dealerships, fund-raising organizations, and telemarketing firms to observe real-life situations of persuasion, Robert B Cialdini Ph.D. found that influence is based on six key principles: reciprocity, commitment and consistency, social proof, authority, liking, scarcity. He later proposed a seventh principle, unity.

Reciprocation: The Old Give and Take … and Take - The rule says that we should try to repay, in kind, what another person has provided us.

Commitment and Consistency: Hobgoblins of the Mind simply, our nearly obsessive desire to be (and to appear) consistent with what we have already done.

Social Proof: Truths Are Us - that one means we use to determine what is correct is to find out what other people think is correct.

Liking: The Friendly Thief – As a rule, we most prefer to say yes to the requests of someone we know and like.

Authority: Directed Deference - a deep-seated sense of duty to authority within us all.

Scarcity: The Rule of the Few - opportunities seem more valuable to us when their availability is limited.

Unity: The more we identify ourselves with other people, the more we are influenced by them.

Cialdini 2007

Undue influence used to overturn a will

A testator, who was divorced after 20 years, remarried and a year later wrote a new will in which he left his entire estate to his second wife, leaving nothing to his two adult children of his first marriage. Under the will, if his second wife were to predecease the testator, her son from her first marriage would take everything and serve as executor of the will. When the second wife was dying the testator visited his lawyer and indicated that he wanted to change his will and leave everything to his own children. He never wrote a new will, however, and died just 4 months after the death of his second wife. Under the testator's will, the son of his second wife inherited everything. The testator's children of his first marriage successfully brought a claim of undue influence based on the acts of the second wife who, knowing that the testator had a morbid fear of divorce (he had attempted suicide after his first divorce), had insisted on his leaving his estate to her and her son or else she might divorce him.

Frolik 2001

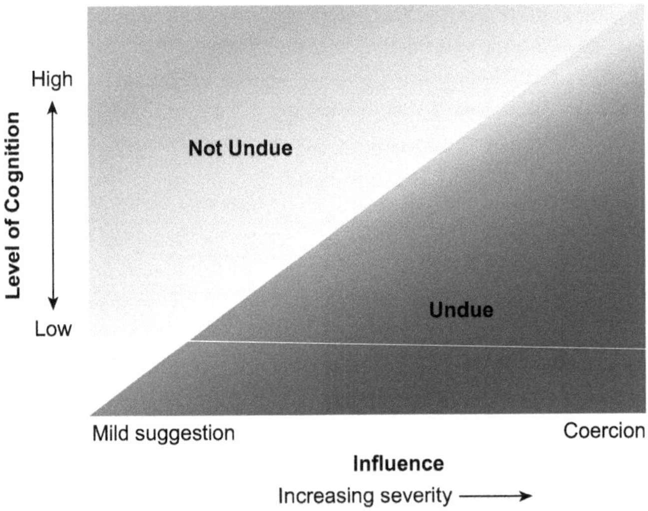

Relationship between cognitive capacity and influence. The lower the capacity or cognitive status of an individual, the less influence would be required to determine that the individual was incapable or unduly influenced. Conversely, an individual with only mild impairment of cognitivefunction would have to be subjected to a severe level of influence to the point to coercion or containment before that influence would be considered undue. *Source: From Shulman, K. I., C. A. Cohen, F. C. Kirsh, I. M. Hull and P. R. Champine (2007). "Assessment of testamentary capacity and vulnerability to undue influence." American Journal of Psychiatry 164(5): 722–727. Reprinted with permission from American Journal of Psychiatry, (Copyright © 2007). American Psychiatric Association. All Rights Reserved.*

Contemporaneous evaluation of undue influence

Geriatric forensic evaluators may become involved in the assessment of testamentary capacity and undue influence when a will is contested by third parties. In these circumstances, family members or other individuals may challenge the will in probate court by claiming that the testator either lacked testamentary capacity at the time the will was executed or was unduly influenced. Assessments of this type may also be required when the issue of guardianship is raised. The ability to make a valid will is one of the capacities which may be assessed along with guardianship statutes, along with the assessment of the individual's capacity to manage his or her financial affairs and make healthcare decisions.

Undue influence on a weakened testator

A 91-year-old testator, confined to a nursing home, signed a new will that favored two of his children over the other two. The trial court had found the testator lacked testamentary capacity and also was the victim of undue influence. On appeal, the court upheld the finding of undue influence. At the time of the execution of the will, the testator suffered from a brain disorder, had a poor memory, was hard of hearing and was disoriented with respect to time, place, and regular activities. According to the court, the "loss of memory and disorientation resulted in [his] relying on other individuals for all his needs and information." The staff at the nursing home testified that the testator was very susceptible to suggestion and influence. The appeals courtheld the will invalid on the grounds of undue influence because, in the opinion of the court, the evidence that the testator was "mentally weak and highly suggestible" when coupled with the evidence of acts of undue influence was sufficient to justify application of the doctrine and overturn the will.

Frolik, 2001

Retrospective evaluation of undue influence

In terms of a deceased or incapacitated testator, clearly, the methodology for the evaluation of testamentary capacity is very different when the assessment is retrospective. This generally occurs when a will is contested after the testator has died, but can also occur under other circumstances.

Changes in the will of a living testator may only come to light years after the changes were made. The testator may now be severely demented and no longer able to provide an account of his or her intentions at the time the will was changed. In such circumstances, an assessment of the individual's current cognitive and emotional status does little to assist the court. In either case, the role of the evaluator is to gather as much information about the testator's cognitive and emotional status at the time the changes were made. It is often necessary to rely on a careful examination of the individual's medical and financial records as well as any other reliable sources of information such as collateral interviews of uninterested parties (Mart, 2016).

Lessons in estate and succession planning

Shakespeare's King Lear is an example of an older adult who use poor judgment in determining how and when to distribute their assets to their children. The opening of King Lear reveals the King's intent to divest his kingdom to his three daughters. Similar to many older adults, he "wishes unburdened to crawl toward death." However, he adds a cruel twist. His three daughters must publicly profess their love for him with "the largest bounty to whoever doth love him most." This was a narcissistic and capricious act with tragic consequences for him and his one sincerely devoted daughter, Cordelia who refused to be hypocritical as were her two older sisters. Leaving himself no control of his assets and putting himself at the mercy of two greedy, ambitious and vindictive daughters, Shakespeare's Lear provides us with a cautionary tale.

Shulman 2018

Conclusion

The world's rapidly growing population of older adults comprises diverse racial, ethnic, gender and sexual orientation, and minority populations. Elder abuse can be expected to increase in the coming years due to demographic trends and other social changes. Much remains to be learned about how to prevent elder abuse and how to intervene effectively.

Adults of all ages strive to maintain dignity and independence, seeking a good, long life free from harm and abuse. Careful elder abuse evaluations are needed to help shine a light on the issues surrounding elder abuse and to serve our vulnerable elderly population. Geriatric forensic evaluators play an important role in the identification of and protection against elder abuse.

Selected references

American Bar Association, 2008. Commission on Law and Aging – American Psychological Association of Older Adults with Diminished Capacity: A Handbook for Psychologists. Available at https://www.apa.org/images/capacity-psychologist-handbook_tcm7-78003.pdf.

Acierno, R., et al., 2010. Prevalence and correlates of emotional, physical, sexual, and financial abuse and potential neglect in the United States: the National Elder Mistreatment Study. Am. J. Public Health 100 (2), 292–297.

Adams, S.D., Lichtenberg, P., April 2014. How to protect and help clients with diminished capacity. MetLife J.

Beach, S.R., Schulz, R., Castle, N.G., Rosen, J., 2010. Financial exploitation and psychological mistreatment among older adults: differences between African Americans and non-African Americans in a population-based survey. Gerontol. 50 (6), 744–757.

Beach, S.R., Carpenter, C.R.M., Rosen, T.M., Sharps, P.P., Gelles, R.P., 2016. Screening and detection of elder abuse: research opportunities and lessons learned from emergency geriatric care, intimate partner violence, and child abuse. J. Elder Abuse Negl. 28 (4–5), 185–216.

CDC, 2018. Elder Abuse: Definitions. From: https://www.cdc.gov/violenceprevention/elderabuse/definitions.html.

Cialdini, R.B., 2007. Influence: The Psychology of Persuasion. Collins: Imprint of HarperCollins, New York, New York.

Connolly, M., 2014. The Elder Justice Roadmap. U. D. o. Justice.

Cooper, C., Selwood, A., Blanchard, M., Walker, Z., Blizard, R., Livingston, G., 2010. The determinants of family caregivers' abusive behaviour to people with dementia: results of the CARD study. J. Affect Disord. 121, 136–142.

Council, N.R., 2003. Elder Mistreatment: Abuse, Neglect, and Exploitation in an Aging America. National Academies Press.

Dong, X. (Ed.), 2017. Elder Abuse: Research, Practice and Policy.

Frolik, L.A., 2001. The strange interplay of testamentary capacity and the doctrine of undue influence. Are we protecting older testators or overriding individual preferences? Int. J. Law Psychiatry 24 (2–3), 253–266.

Holzer, J., Kohn, R., Ellison, J., Recupero, P. (Eds.), 2018. Geriatric Forensic Psychiatry: Principles and Practice. Oxford University Press, Oxford, UK.

Kosberg, J.I., Garcia, J.L., 1995. Elder Abuse: International and Cross-Cultural Perspectives.

Lichtenberg, P.A., 2016. Financial exploitation, financial capacity, and Alzheimer's disease. Am. Psychol. 71 (4), 312.

Mart, E.G., 2016. Neuropsychological assessment of testamentary capacity and undue influence. Arch. Clin. Neuropsychol. 31 (6), 554–561.

The MetLife Study of Elder Financial Abuse Crimes of Occasion, June 2011. Desperation, and Predation Against America's Elders. Available at https://ltcombudsman.org/uploads/files/issues/mmi-elder-financial-abuse.pdf.

Navarro, A.E., Gassoumis, Z.D., Wilber, K.H., 2013. Holding abusers accountable: an elder abuse forensic center increases criminal prosecution of financial exploitation. Gerontol. 53 (2), 303–312.

Reis, M., Nahmiash, D., 1998. Validation of the indicators of abuse (IOA) screen. Gerontologist 38, 471–480.

Roberto, K.A., 2016. The complexities of elder abuse. Am. Psychol. 71 (4), 302.

Shields, L., Hunsaker, D., Hunsaker, J., 2004. Abuse and neglect: a ten-year review of mortality and morbidity in our elderly in a large metropolitan area. J. Forensic Sci. 49 (1), 122–127.

Shulman, K.I., Cohen, C.A., Kirsh, F.C., Hull, I.M., Champine, P.R., 2007. Assessment of testamentary capacity and vulnerability to undue influence. Am. J. Psychiatry 164 (5), 722–727.
Shulman, K., 2018. All about Estates - Blog Posts 2014-2016. From. https://www.allaboutestates.ca/author/kshulman/.
Terra Nova Films, 2012. He Wouldn't Turn Me Loose: The Sexual Abuse Case of 96-Year-Old Miss Mary. From. https://www.psychotherapy.net/video/social-work-elder-sexual-abuse.
Wilber, K.H., Reynolds, S.L., 1997. Introducing a framework for defining financial abuse of the elderly. J. Elder Abuse Negl. 8 (2), 61–80.
Wood, S., Rakela, B., Liu, P.J., Navarro, A.E., Bernatz, S., Wilber, K.H., Homier, D., 2014. Neuropsychological profiles of victims of financial elder exploitation at the los angeles county elder abuse forensic center. J. Elder Abuse & Neglect. 26 (4), 414–423.
Wood, S., Liu, P.-J., 2012. Undue influence and financial capacity: a clinical perspective. Generations 36 (2), 53–58.

CHAPTER SIX

Geriatric forensic report writing and testimony

Contents

The Clinician's Guide to Geriatric Forensic Evaluations
ISBN: 978-0-12-815034-4
https://doi.org/10.1016/B978-0-12-815034-4.00006-4

Forensic psychiatric reports and testimony are critical tool for geriatric psychiatric clinicians serving the court as experts. Developing skills in report writing will help geriatric forensic clinicians take the lead in helping the court understand psychiatric conditions in older people.

Testifying is not the most common activity of geriatric forensic clinicians – report writing is. Most civil cases settle prior to trial, so court testimony is relatively rare. For the most part, the clinicians' contribution in an expert role will be in the form of a formal report. A written report of a psychiatric evaluation, incorporating the expert's findings, often serves as the basis for the settlement or resolution of a case, much more often than psychiatric expert testimony.

This chapter will review some of the key considerations for geriatric forensic clinicians and preparing geriatric forensic reports and testimony during depositions or trials. Distinguished authors in the field of forensic psychiatry have offered a lot of valuable guidance on these issues. The reader is encouraged to consult the seminal texts listed below established texts for further detail and guidance.

Key resources on geriatric forensic report writing and testimony

1. Babitsky, S., & Mangraviti, J. J. (2002). Writing and defending your expert report: The step by step guide with models. MA: SEAK, Inc.
2. Buchanan, A. and M. A. Norko (2011). The Psychiatric Report: Principles and Practice of Forensic Writing, Cambridge University Press.
3. Gutheil, TJ (2009). The psychiatrist as expert witness. American Psychiatric Publishing, Inc.
4. Gutheil, TJ (2007). Practical Approaches to Forensic Mental Health Testimony, Wolters Kluwer.
5. Reid, W. H. (2013). Developing a Forensic Practice: Operations and Ethics for Experts, Routledge.
6. Soliman, S & Resnick PJ: Geriatric Forensic Report Writing. In Holzer et al. GERIATRIC FORENSIC PSYCHIATRY: Principles and Practice. Oxford University Press, 2018.

Ethical considerations for forensic reports

To summarize some of the unique issues that arise in geriatric forensic psychiatry cases, the following table reminds us of ethical considerations for forensic reports. Resnick and Soliman summarized ethical considerations that apply to forensic reports and testimony, based on The American Academy of Psychiatry and the Law's Ethical Guidelines for the Practice of Forensic Psychiatry.

Ethical considerations

Qualifications

- Ensure that your skills, experience, expertise qualify to address issues in referral
- Report qualifications accurately
- Avoid using self-aggrandizing comments
- Attach psychologist's report if you lack expertise in interpreting tests
- State factors clearly that limit your ability to form a complete and accurate opinion
- State the reason for the information unavailable
- Explain the steps you took to seek the information
- Note the portions of your opinion that may be affected by the missing data

Informed consent

- Informed consent must be knowing, voluntary, and competent
- Advise the evaluee of the nature of the evaluation
- Inform evaluees if they do participate in the evaluation
- If person lacks capacity, obtain consent from a surrogate decision-maker, guardian

Confidentiality

- It is important to hold in confidence information learned during evaluation, treatment
- An individual must be informed of the limits of confidentiality
- Avoid unnecessary disclosure of confidential information

Objectivity

- Forensic psychiatrists must accurately report all relevant information
- Prepare a report only if the attorney desires one
- Resist the unconscious temptation to support the retaining attorney's position
- Avoid serving in a dual role
- If you cannot avoid a dual role, inform the patient of your dual role.
- Resist pressure of being treated as a part of "the team" by attorneys.
- Correspondence with the retaining attorney should be professional & objective.

Soliman and Resnick, 2018

Geriatric forensic report writing

Skill at report writing is one of the defining skills in geriatric forensic practice. Geriatric forensic reports provide the court with a lasting record of your opinions and the basis for those opinions. Roles of the forensic report include communicating information, analyzing, interpreting and communicating clinical data into forensic opinions, which prepare the groundwork for potential future testimony. Report writing usually involves answering specific legal questions posed by attorneys.

A good report will help you focus your opinions and make it easier to prepare for testimony if that is required. Some jurisdictions may require a formal report before a lawsuit can proceed.

Quality reports are an important tool for resolving cases, often contributing to settlements in civil cases or plea negotiations in a criminal context. The geriatric forensic report may affect the outcome of the case, with profound consequences for an elder's life and livelihood.

Workflow

The forensic expert's preparation for the report begins as soon as expert receives a consultation request from an attorney. The expert should obtain details about the legal question, deadlines and other important information about the case.

Whenever possible, allocate ample time for reviewing records and drafting your report. Though retaining attorneys may work on relatively short deadlines and request a report within a short time frame, report writing should not be excessively rushed or delayed until the last minute. It is worth taking the time to do an exemplary job with each psychiatric report, because the document will become a lasting record once submitted.

There is no rigid set of rules for report preparation. Nevertheless, a routine approach to the forensic report, akin to a clinical interview outline or template, can help guide the expert and serve as a type of scaffolding for the expert's future involvement. However, clinicians should tailor their approach to suit the case at hand.

Brodsky's maxims to help expert witnesses prepare for testimony and cross-examination

- Review current literature on the topic about which you will testify
- Witnesses often feel like aliens in the courtroom so consider going into the empty courtroom alone and sitting for a while or sitting in on other trials.

Brodsky's maxims to help expert witnesses prepare for testimony and cross-examination (*cont'd*)

- Meet with the attorney prior to the direct examination and be involved in preparing the questions
- Prepare a list of professionally relevant and complete qualifying questions for the attorney to use in the opening of the direct examination
- If you make a mistake during testimony, correct the error as soon as you can. If you cannot, let it go

ABA/APA, 2008

Best practices

Only write a report if retaining counsel requests it

Reports are usually requested by the retaining attorney, but sometimes may be requested by a court. If your opinions do not support the case of the attorney who retained you, that attorney will be unlikely to request a report, since a report could be harmful to the case.

Geriatric forensic reports will likely become available to the other side's lawyer, and possibly a judge or jury. It is important that a clinician does not write forensic report unless the retaining entity, other attorney or the court, requests it.

Attorneys hate surprises. Do not write a report unless specifically requested by retaining counsel or by the court.

Follow a usual routine or protocol

As with clinical work, there are few rigid rules about how to accomplish the complex tasks of geriatric forensic practice. Clinicians must follow their professional judgment in their forensic activities. Nevertheless, it is advisable for clinicians to establish a basic routine or protocol for report preparation, and to take the time to follow it when appropriate.

It is advisable to accept cases only when you will have enough time to properly prepare for the case, review materials and render opinions. Doing things in a hurry may lead to the result being sloppy or incomplete, and could cause embarrassment later.

You may find it valuable to collect and file together specific documents for each case that you are working on, including a signed contract or retention agreement, a statement from the attorney describing the requested services, the legal complaint and responses and information about the legal standard to be applied in the case.

Identify the legal issue and any relevant legal standards

Be sure to know the relevant legal standard that applies in the case. For example, for a case of alleged undue influence, you should know how that concepts are defined in that specific jurisdiction. In a guardianship case, the legal issues include functioning level, so that should be specifically addressed in the report.

Use relevant legal terms correctly. Specific legal terms of arts include words or phrases that have a very specific legal meaning. Some of these are included in the table below (Reid, 2013).

Legal terms and phrases with definitions that may vary across jurisdictions

- Reasonable medical/psychiatric certainty/probability
- Competence (competency)
- Know
- Appreciate
- Undue influence
- Testamentary capacity
- Standard of care
- Responsibility
- Foreseeability
- Cause (causation)
- Negligent (negligence); gross negligence

Reid, 2013

Knowing the precise definitions of legal terms of art is outside the scope of the geriatric psychiatrists' training and expertize, so clinicians should not be afraid to ask the lawyer whether or not they are using a term correctly. If in doubt, consider getting your own legal dictionary, rather than just googling terms.

Recommended legal dictionary

Black's Law Dictionary, 10th Edition, Bryan A. Garner, Ed. Thomson West, 2014.

Ideally, your report will have a specific section devoted to an assessment of the relevant legal criteria pertaining to the forensic issue. For example, a testamentary capacity report could include the specific questions you asked about the legal elements of testamentary capacity.

Write in a clear style

To be helpful in assisting the court, geriatric forensic reports must first be clear and understandable to the reader. Reports should be concise and jargon-free.

Tips for a clear writing style

- Aim for an understandable "storytelling" style
- Each report should be a self-contained document
- Start with the most important information, stating the general before the specific.
- Introduce key individuals before discussing them
- Aim to write your report while the source material is still fresh in your mind
- Write for an educated lay audience, not your professional peers

Soliman and Resnick (2018) outline four fundamental principles of good writing: [1] clarity, [2] simplicity, [3] brevity and [4] humanity. Clinicians who want to produce high-quality forensic reports should adhere to these basic principles of good writing.

Style guidance

For timeless English writing and style guidance, an excellent guide is the classic *Strunk and White's Elements of Style*. If offers direct guidance on rules of structure and making the written word as clear and understandable as possible.

Recommended style guide

Strunk and White, Elements of Style 1999

In terms of length, short is generally preferable to long, sticking to the point as much as possible (Strunk and White, 2000). Have the report answer specific questions. Extraneous material can be distracting or harmful to the case. Short reports often take extra thought and care, and can actually taking longer to write than a lengthy report. It can be challenging to distill the important facts from a large mass of information reviewed.

Avoiding hedge words

"Hedging" or mitigating words such as "apparently" and "possibly" lessen the impact of your writing. They imply uncertainty and weaken your report, indicating that you are guessing about the facts or are imprecize in citing a source of information. It is better to avoid hedge words.

Instead, simply state the source of your information, perhaps providing a citation to the record for reference. Your opinions must be stated with reasonable medical certainty. In most jurisdictions, this means "more likely than not."

"Hedging" language to avoid

- I think
- It appears that
- In a sense
- Apparently
- Possibly
- Supposedly
- Reportedly

Babitsky and Mangraviti, 2002

Editing and proofreading

A report full of errors makes a poor impression and invites questions about your competence in reaching your conclusions. Prior to submission, be sure to review your report for grammatical and typographical errors. You will also want to review the content and organization of the report, to be sure that it fulfills its purpose and follows a logical format. It is sometimes helpful to have a colleague read over the report. Verb tenses should accurately reflect the time an event occurred. It is best to use the past tense, for events that occurred in the past. Omit unnecessary material. Poor or erroneous vocabulary could get you or the case into trouble. The language of the legal arena is often very specific, with definitions sometimes differing from ordinary lay usage of terms, including fact or reasonable certainty. It is sometimes helpful to have a colleague read over the report.

Types of Proofreading

- Substance Proofreading: for organization, data, and the logical consistency of your opinion.
- Style Proofreading: for sentence structure, correct word choice, omitting of unnecessary material.
- Keyboard Proofreading: for typographical errors and incorrect grammar.

Soliman and Resnick, 2018

The final product

Remember that your report is representative of you and your work, and can affect future referrals and your professional reputation. The final report should provide enough information to allow the reader to fully understand your opinions and the bases for your opinions.

Qualities of a great geriatric forensic report

- Standalone document
- Concise, with short sentences and paragraphs
- Properly formatted
- Clearly organized, user friendly
- Contains everything required
- Opinions separate from facts
- Carefully and clearly worded
- Excellent grammar and spelling
- Very neat

Organize the report

In general, reports should be organized to address the specific forensic issue. However, the format and style vary with case, jurisdiction and expert. Consider using a template for guidance, but do not produce boilerplate reports. Always tailor your report to the specific referral issue. Organize your report to address the forensic question at hand in this particular case.

Several sources have valuable templates, particularly Reid's excellent and practical volume, incorporating useful styles and content.

Recommended templates to help organize your report

- Reid, W. H. (2013). Developing a Forensic Practice: Operations and Ethics for Experts, Routledge.
- Berger, S. H. (2008). "Template for quickly creating forensic psychiatry reports." J Am Acad Psychiatry Law 36(3): 388–392.

Possible disclaimers/caveats

- Your report is preliminary
- You assume records received are reasonably representative of the overall facts
- If additional information is obtained about the case, you reserve the right to amend your report or add to it
- Your opinions were formed using the procedures and information customarily relied upon by colleagues in similar cases
- Whether or not you actually examined the relevant persons, and if not, whether or not an adequate examination might change your opinions

Reid, 2013

Creating an outline can be useful and can force you to think about the structure of your report, what information you will include, your opinion and supporting facts. Planning the appropriate structure will help you achieve clarity in your report. Subdividing a report into categories will make it more accessible to the reader.

Know the specific facts of the case

As you gather relevant data for review prior to writing a report, compile a list of all your sources of information. It is often helpful to organize this data with a numbered list, including correspondence, depositions, reports and other information sources. Seek out any missing information. In cases with voluminous records, it can be difficult to keep track of numerous evaluations, family members or events over time. Creating charts and family trees can help you stay organized and on top of the facts. For retrospective evaluations, consider creating a timeline of key events to include in your report.

Provide citations for literature pertaining to this specific case. Be sure to use current versions of textbooks and the Diagnostic and Statistical Manual.

Throughout your report, you should clearly separate factual data from your professional opinions or conclusions. The latter belong only in your Opinion section.

Offer opinions only if supported by data

The Opinion section is the most important section in a geriatric forensic report. It should be carefully planned. Opinions should flow logically from the data, and not go beyond it. Review each piece of evidence to be sure there is a factual basis for it and that it actually supports your specific opinion.

Opinions should generally be expressed to a reasonable degree of medical certainty. Each of your opinions should be accompanied by reasonable explanation. It should not contain facts that have not been included in the body of your report. Start with the key opinions, then list supporting facts for each point. List the facts supporting your opinions in order of strongest to weakest.

Problems and pitfalls

Acting like an attorney

Forensic clinicians should bear in mind their duty to be objective and assist the court in finding the truth. As an expert in geriatric forensic psychiatry, it is not your job to advocate for the retaining party. Attorneys are retained to be advocates for clients, but experts should not be advocates. Avoid language in your reports and correspondence that suggests you are biased. Your opinions should be based on the facts of the case, not on discussions with the retaining attorney.

Ethical expert witnesses are impartial and unbiased.

Though you may want to discuss the report format or legal questions with the lawyer, even helpful ways to frame your opinions, do not let a lawyer write your report. Your opinions should be based on your independent review of the facts. Do not insert opinions that are not your own genuine opinions based on your independent review of the records and your own understanding of the case. Your report must never misrepresent the overall case.

Be cautious about using legal terms including the words "legally" or "legal", since a skilled cross-examiner may then ask you the precise legal definition of such terms. Stick to the psychiatric issues you are qualified to address.

It can be appropriate for retaining counsel to review an expert's draft report for proofreading purposes, such as catching factual errors, wrong assumptions or inadvertent omissions. However, be alert to any pressure to change your opinions. As an expert, you must be objective, maintaining independence and integrity. You should not take on an advocacy role.

Confusing clinical and forensic reports

The purpose and structure of a clinical report differs from that of a forensic report. Do not list clinical findings the way you would at medical rounds. Instead, start with the referral issue and organize your report to best address that issue, tailoring the sections of the report around it. Look beyond the data to create a coherent narrative based on the information you have gathered from the various sources.

Your report should contain logical arguments supported by the facts of the case, presented in an objective manner. Depending on the forensic question at hand, you may want to include in your diagnostic section that you specifically considered the possibility of malingering.

Tailor your report to the specific legal questions being asked.

As in clinical settings, respect for persons should be maintained. In a forensic context, this may mean taking steps to protect the evaluee's privacy by excluding details which may be pertinent from a clinical perspective, unless they pertain to the legal question being asked. For example, elements of developmental history (bedwetting in childhood) or sexual history (promiscuity or age of first intercourse) may add little to the evaluation and should be excluded to avoid embarrassing the evaluee unnecessarily.

In forensic reports, consider referring to everyone by the appropriate prefix, Mr., Ms. or Dr. followed by their surname. Avoid using generic terms such as "the testator" or "the defendant" since such terms can seem dehumanizing, as if the report were about a generic product rather than a human being.

Equating dementia with lack of capacity

Geriatric forensic examiners should be mindful to avoid unfounded links between diagnostic and legal conclusions. Dementia does not automatically equate lack of testamentary capacity. You should have a factual basis for opinions, and not simply leap from a diagnosis to a forensic psychiatric opinion. For example, while dementia may explain cognitive deficits relevant to testamentary capacity, such as a testatrix's difficulty remembering the extent of her assets, the dementia itself does not equal lack of testamentary capacity.

Dementia does not automatically equate with lack of testamentary capacity.

Addressing the wrong forensic issue

Forensic clinicians should generally avoid answering questions that were not asked, among them the ultimate issue: the legal issue being addressed by the trier-of-fact. It is better to phrase your conclusions in the language of the legal test being considered.

Be sure to adequately address the relevant legal issues.

Getting distracted by family dynamics

The role of collateral information is key in geriatric forensic evaluations, but fraught with difficulty. Family conflict has ramifications for both the clinical and the medico-legal practice. In cases of dementia, conflict may be based on accusations of inadequate care, financial exploitation (either through control of money or manipulation of a will) and/or failure to communicate with other family members or sequestration of the person with dementia (Peisah et al., 2006). Tensions in the family often run high in the context of geriatric forensic issues, and it is critical that experts avoid getting distracted by family dynamics.

Relying on unsubstantiated diagnoses and inaccurate data

Seek additional records if you notice inaccurate or missing data in the data provided by retaining counsel. Clarify data sources. On a related note, do not submit an inaccurate CV.

Disregarding data that conflicts with opinion

In forming opinions about a forensic case, experts should be careful not to ignore disconfirming data. Psychiatrists may be asked to omit information, but this could weaken the credibility of the report and raise questions about their ethics. Experts should also be mindful to avoid errors of omission such as leaving out key details, oversimplifying the story and/or persuading with a biased report to favor one side. All of which would misrepresent the facts of the case to the court, and create bias in an effort to meet attorney demands.

Misapplying psychological testing

Geriatric forensic evaluations for cognitive concerns often involve psychological or neuropsychological testing. Discussion of the neuropsychological testing in the report should note any irregularities in test administration, such as a break during a timed test or uncooperativeness, If the testing was completed by a psychologist, consider quoting their report or put it in an appendix in your own report. Discuss how you considered this data in forming your opinion. Generally, psychological tests do not directly address the forensic issue at hand. Avoid jumping from test results to an illogical forensic psychiatric conclusion or opinion.

Ignoring the dynamic nature of capacity

Cognitive impairments may be due to reversible causes including delirium, medication side effects and others. Be careful not to project too far into the future, based on a snapshot of someone's functioning, i.e. a delirious elder with cognitive impairment undergoing guardianship proceedings.

Decision making capacity in older people can change over time, and should be monitored and reassessed as needed.

Capacity is dynamic. It is important to consider reversible causes, especially delirium, before making long-term decisions. In a medically ill geriatric population, cognition can fluctuate, and capacity can fluctuate dramatically over time.

Destroying records too soon

As with clinical treatment records, forensic psychiatric files should be maintained according to professional guidelines. The content of a forensic file differs from a clinical treatment file. Forensic files can become part of legal proceedings, beginning with the initial contact from the referring attorney or courts. Copies of phone notes, letters and other correspondence should be retained, along with the timesheets tracking the days and hours spent for forensic activities related to the case. The records may involve interviews of the client and collateral, review of records, travel records and others. After a case is completed, the expert can inquire to see whether the referring attorney would like to have the available documents returned or shredded. Information disclosed as evidence during a trial becomes part of the public record.

Your forensic file can become part of the legal proceedings, and you can be asked to testify about verbal communications with retaining counsel.

Oral communications with the attorneys are one way to keep them private. Various rules may apply that require you to divulge what you discussed with the attorney and what was in report drafts etc. However, you should keep records that document key facts. For unrecorded phone calls with the retaining counsel or others, you may still be required to testify about these oral communications—rendering even those also discoverable as long as you remember when asked.

You are not generally required to keep previous versions of files as long as you type over them in the usual course of your work. Nevertheless, if you are subpoenaed, most jurisdictions will require you to produce any drafts or notes. Do not destroy copies of anything you have sent to the attorney, including drafts. In fact, do not destroy anything related to the case once your records have been subpoenaed. Retaining counsel can likely advise you about what you must produce when subpoenaed. You may want to discuss that with the lawyer who retained you. Certain things may indeed not be discoverable or not need to be provided to the other side when subpoenaed.

Avoid labeling the report a "draft," a "work product," or "confidential" since this will alert the cross-examiner to the fact that there are or were other versions of your report. It can also be made to look like you are trying to hide something from the opposing party or from the court (Babitsky and Mangraviti, 2002).

Geriatric forensic testimony

If testifying in a deposition, your depositions will almost always be civil "discovery" depositions—a chance for the other side to learn what you will say in court.

Deposition testimony has the same weight as trial testimony. There are strict rules about the process of deposition. Others may be present including retained opposing lawyers, a court reporter as well as other consultants, occasionally the litigants and others.

You may receive a subpoena duces tecum from the opposing lawyer, i.e. a demand to attend and bring your records, files, billing materials, etc. Trial is relatively rare.

Best practices

As with the preceding section, these "best practices" are not to be understood as a standard of practice. There may be fair variations in actual forensic context and clinicians should use their professional judgment applied to the particular case at hand.

Be aware of deposition and trial dates

Depositions are scheduled by the lawyer and can usually accommodate your schedule. Trials are less flexible, since they are a complex process controlled by the judge orchestrating it. You must be available for any dates you have agreed to in advance. However, in civil cases particularly, which tend to be the most common in geriatric forensic psychiatry, the majority of trial dates will be changed, or the case will be resolved before trial.

Prepare with retaining counsel

Do not simply show up at court to testify, but instead hold a pre-testimony conference with the retaining attorney so he/she can bring you up to date about the case, go over likely questions, review what he/she thinks is important, give advice and help you prepare for direct and cross examination. Consider formulating some answers to standard questions in advance.

You will be asked about your background, and other common questions about your field. You can set limits on irrelevant personal questions that do not pertain to the subject matter of the case. It is ultimately the judge's decision whether or not something is irrelevant, so be prepared for that. Avoid sharing your social security number, home address, or personal number since much testimony is public information.

Tell the truth

Experts must tell the truth. Honesty and objectivity are one of the hallmarks of an ethical forensic psychiatrist (AAPL, 2005). Paul Appelbaum notes that this includes both the common view of honesty, i.e., saying what one believes, as well as a proactive duty to avoid the sin of omission by volunteering information that allows one's data and conclusions to be more accurately interpreted. These can be thought of as "subjective" and "objective" truths, summarized by the table below (Buchanan and Norko, 2011).

The truth, the whole truth...

Subjective truth-telling

- Resembles the common view of honesty, i.e., saying what one believes
- Expert does not hold one opinion but express another because doing so will bring financial gain, avoid embarrassment, or win admiration

Objective truth-telling

- Placing the conclusions of a report in a sufficient context that the reader is not misled into believing something that is likely untrue
- Proactive duty to avoid a sin of omission by volunteering information that allows one's data and conclusions to be more accurately interpreted
- Includes noting the limitations of one's evaluation (e.g., lack of sufficient time, absence of important records, uncooperativeness of the evaluee, one's own inexperience) and their consequences for the certainty with which one can state one's opinion
- Encompasses limitations on scientific knowledge that may preclude definitive answers to a question or make even the best assessments inherently tentative

Paul Appelbaum, in Buchanan and Norko, 2011

Money, or attention from a high-profile case and media coverage, may be motivating factors when it comes to influencing a psychiatric report. In addition, the psychiatrist may have strong moral or political opinions about the case, compromising objectivity. Experts should be mindful about potential influences and sources of bias for their opinions and clinical activities. It may be helpful to consult an experienced colleague who can offer objective advice.

The expert who cannot afford to walk away from a case is the one at greatest risk of having his/her integrity compromised.

Speak clearly and simply

Your geriatric forensic testimony will usually consist of answering questions, not giving lectures. Listen carefully to the questions and be clear and firm with your answers. Avoid answering too quickly, and aim to give short, direct answers to the questions being asked. Do not answer more than was asked.

Look credible and professional

Think about your role and purpose in court, and dress appropriately. Your aim is to appear credible and professional in the eyes of the judge and jury. Consider the impression and impact on your credibility of your clothing, jewelry and personal grooming. Avoid distracting the judge and jury from your opinions and professional credibility. Styles are constantly changing and evolving, and like so much else in medicine and forensic psychiatry, the final determination is left to your professional judgment. You may want to err on the conservative side, depending on the type of case and jurisdiction where you are called to testify.

Problems and pitfalls

Being a professor, not a teacher

Your testimony will generally consist of answering questions and explaining key concepts in layperson's terms, not giving complicated lectures. Think middle school teacher, not distinguished professor.

Anger and defensiveness

Avoid getting ruffled by cross examination or making snide comments about the parties or opposing experts, since this will diminish your credibility as a forensic expert. It is acceptable to disagree with experts for the other side and respectfully to criticize their methods. However, refrain from personal attacks and sarcastic or condescending language. Being argumentative will weaken your testimony. Be respectful to everyone.

Avoid partisan arguments and aim for unbiased expert opinion. Simply state your opinions with reasonable medical certainty, and list the reasons supporting your opinions. If you discuss your disagreements with other experts, refrain from any personal attacks or condescending language. Instead, specify the areas of disagreement and list the evidence supporting your opinion.

Be mentally prepared to have your credibility laity questioned, including past trial and deposition testimony, licensing and hospital privilege status, references to you on the Internet and your writings. Questions about your credibility are an expected part of expert testimony. Actually, your credibility may be more likely to be called into question if the facts strongly support your interpretation, as a tactic or strategy, if the other side cannot refute your opinions.

Be able to tolerate criticism. This is neither a collegial process nor a scientific one. It is not quite "inquisitor," but it is adversarial. You should not be an adversary yourself, but you must tolerate questioning from lawyers who vigorously oppose the side for which you are testifying and who may be very good at turning your words, opinions, and even behaviors to their own advantage.

Do not be alarmed if the opposing lawyer appears frustrated or irritated. Keep your cool and be polite. The lawyer for whom you are testifying will intervene if necessary. Don't take it personally and avoid offering rejoinders or verbose explanations.

Awkwardness about fees

Questions about fees are to be expected in deposition or trial. Experts should not be surprised or defensive about this. Before declining to answer questions about compensation or fees, wait for the lawyer for whom you are testifying to object. The questions may be legitimate. It is fair to ask how much you charge in this case. However, it may or may not be fair to ask how much you made last year in your forensic practice, or what your gross income was last year, unless the judge requires you to answer.

Skeletons in the closet

Experts should be aware that opposing counsel will be motivated to seek any skeletons in your closet. For relatively minor issues such as a past failed attempt on a licensing exam, or a past malpractice lawsuit, it is best to assume a relatively nonchalant stance and avoid getting defensive or ruffled. More serious issues such as criminal convictions, license revocations, controversial past writings or being disqualified on a past expert witness assignment should be discussed in advance with retaining counsel since they may indeed be deal breakers for credible expert testimony.

The "primrose path" and other traps

Listen carefully to each question. Avoid the "primrose path" phenomenon of rapid-fire easy questions with a surprise kicker at the end. Don't try to figure out the opposing lawyer's strategy or to "outsmart" him/her. Don't try to bluff or get outside your expertize. Assume the opposing lawyer knows the answer to every question he/she is asking (especially at trial).

Try to answer questions only once. Lawyers often ask the same question several times, then choose the most advantageous answer. If you don't know an answer, say so. Don't let them talk you out of what you believe to be accurate and appropriate answers. "Is that all your opinions, Doctor?" is a common question. Simply say that you aren't sure what you'll be asked at trial, so you don't know what your answers will be, and you'll be happy to answer any questions the opposing lawyer wishes to ask now. Reserve the possibility of forming new opinions if additional information becomes available.

On a related note, lawyers may demand that you answer yes or no, but ignore this demand if the question cannot reasonably be answered by yes or no, i.e., if that would misconstrue your meaning, and explain why. If the judge says he must answer yes or no, try to explain. However, you may not succeed. The retaining lawyer will have a chance to clarify later. "I don't know," or "I can't answer the question that was asked," are quite acceptable.

Alternatives to "yes or no"

- I don't know
- I can't accurately answer the question yes or no as you phrased it
- Answering yes or no would misconstrue my opinion for the jury or judge
- I don't understand your question

Reid, 2013

Not a memory test

Testimony is not a memory test. Prepare well enough to testify primarily from memory, but ask to refer to notes or records if necessary. Many experts choose not to carry anything to the witness stand except perhaps copies of their reports and/or depositions. If you do take your notes or file to the stand, consider making an extra copy in advance to give it to the opposing lawyer if he or she asks to see what you're referring to during testimony. Taking the expert's notes is an old lawyer trick. You don't want to have to beg to get them back in order to consult them.

Rambling

Testimony is a stepwise process. Avoid answering questions beyond what was asked and don't say anything you can't support. If you cannot support each of your opinions and statements, your conclusions are unlikely to stand up in court.

Stick to your forensic opinions. Open-ended questions may invite you to talk, but be aware that opposing lawyers will be listening for anything in your verbose presentation that they can find which can be turned to their advantage. Simply answer the question, tell the truth concisely and remember the context and environment of your testimony. Answer only what is asked. Be cautious about volunteering answers to unasked questions, and don't over explain your answers. Off-the-cuff explanations may give undeserved information to the other side.

Conclusion

Writing quality forensic reports and being aware of the various implications and consequences of forensic report writing Quality geriatric forensic reports serve not only the individual practitioner and the legal marketplace, but also the mental health profession as a whole. Skilled peer review of your work by more senior colleagues willing to share their expertise can be invaluable as you build your forensic practice.

Selected references

American Academy of Psychiatry and Law Governing Council, 2005. Ethics Guidelines for the Practice of Forensic Psychiatry. The American Academy of Psychiatry and Law. http://www.aapl.org/ethics.htm.

American Bar Association and America Psychological Association, 2008. Assessment of Older Adults with Diminished Capacity: A Handbook for Psychologists. ABA/APA, Washington, DC.

Babitsky, S., Mangraviti, J.J., 2002. Writing and Defending Your Expert Report: The Step by Step Guide with Models. SEAK, Inc, MA.

Berger, S.H., 2008. Template for quickly creating forensic psychiatry reports. J. Am. Acad. Psychiatry Law 36 (3), 388–392.

Buchanan, A., Norko, M.A., 2011. The Psychiatric Report: Principles and Practice of Forensic Writing. Cambridge University Press.

Gutheil, T., 2009. The Psychiatrist as Expert Witness. American Psychiatric Publishing, Inc.

Gutheil, T.J., 2007. Practical Approaches to Forensic Mental Health Testimony. Wolters Kluwer.

Peisah, C., Brodaty, H., Quadrio, C., 2006. Family conflict in dementia: prodigal sons and black sheep. Int. J. Geriatr. Psychiatry 21 (5), 485–492.

Reid, W.H., 2013. Developing a Forensic Practice: Operations and Ethics for Experts. Routledge.

Soliman, S., Resnick, P.J., 2018. Geriatric forensic report writing. In: Holzer, J.C., Kohn, R., Ellison, J.M., Recupero, P.R. (Eds.), Geriatric Forensic Psychiatry: Principles and Practice. Oxford University Press.

Strunk, W., White, E.B., 2000. The Elements of Style, fourth ed. Longman.

Afterword

Growing need for evaluators

As the global population ages, we are seeing a growing need for geriatric forensic evaluations. Increasing rates of dementia and other neurocognitive disorders in the aging population complicate the evaluation and treatment of a growing number of individuals. We are simultaneously facing a critical shortage of medical and mental health professionals with specialized expertise in geriatric forensic evaluations.

Stakes are often high for geriatric forensic evaluees, since finding of incapacity can strip an individual of his or her individual rights.

There is a growing need for geriatric forensic evaluations.

Clinicians working with elderly patients are frequently asked to evaluate capacity and other medicolegal questions. A recent article by Doron et al. in International Psychogeriatrics gives us a fascinating glimpse into the wide range of legal issues where dementia is relevant: legal questions that go far beyond capacity and guardianship issues.

Contests of wills and trusts are increasing in common law jurisdictions around the world. We will soon be facing an unprecedented transfer of personal wealth amassed by the Baby Boomer generation. Assessment for testamentary capacity and vulnerability to undue influence can be complex. It often requires retrospective evaluation of a deceased testator. For allegations of undue influence, there is active debate within the field about whether psychiatrists should attempt to answer the ultimate legal question (Plotkin et al., 2016).

Many tools and instruments have been proposed to assist clinicians with geriatric forensic evaluations. These include specialized instruments for medical decision making and for financial capacity assessment. Such tools can potentially be helpful; however, none are currently in widespread use.

Emerging areas of research, future directions of the field

Needs of older offenders

The forensic issues among older adults and the psychiatric care of the elderly in the criminal justice system are becoming a major public health concern. A major overhaul of all the systems that care for these vulnerable individuals is needed now (Tampi et al., 2018).

The psychiatric care of the elderly in the criminal justice system is becoming a major public health concern.

Mental health and general medical care for older adults requires specific on-site or consultation expertise in geriatric medicine and psychiatry, as well as potential changes in infrastructure, both of which may be prohibitively expensive. However, compassionate and effective treatment of older prisoners requires that prison and legal systems facilitate this expert care. To address this situation, strategic revisions of the criminal justice system are needed to alleviate prison overcrowding and consequent inadequate medical care for inmates, especially the elder ones. The unique, age-related demands of this older population predict an increased need for forensic psychiatrists with a thorough knowledge and expertise in geriatrics, as more forensic psychiatric evaluations will be needed before trial in both civil and criminal cases, during incarceration, and at the time of parole (Yarnell et al., 2017).

Criminalization of elder abuse

The field is moving toward the criminalization of elder abuse, and especially with the passage of the Elder Abuse Prevention and Prosecution Act of 2017, which was signed October 18th, 2018. Forensic interviewing is going to become increasingly important.

The field is moving toward the criminalization of elder abuse.

Improving work with multidisciplinary teams

Forensic interviews are best conducted within the context of a multidisciplinary team. In the future, there will be a need to continue intensive collaboration and find better ways to work together, including all of the stakeholders.

Multidisciplinary approach for geriatric forensic evaluations:

- Persons who report elder abuse
- Law enforcement personnel
- Emergency Medical Personnel
- Family, neighbors, friends
- Adult protective services
- Prosecuting and Defending attorneys
- Judges
- Mental health professionals
- Medical providers
- Facility staff, and
- Financial institutions.

Forensic interviews are best conducted within the context of a multidisciplinary team.

Cultural issues

What is cultural competence?

Building an awareness of one's own culture.
Expanding one's cultural imagination.
Becoming informed of various cultural beliefs and practices.
Developing intercultural skills of observation and communication.
Incorporating cultural interpretation into reports and testimonies.

Holzer et al., 2018

Working with the elderly may pose challenges, since age brings another dimension to the cultural element. Whereas an assessment across different cultures and different languages generally takes longer than a comparable assessment without these barriers, an older individual, who could have a dementing illness and other medical problems, may require additional interviews and further collateral information. Older individuals are also more likely to be established in their points of view and slower or more resistant to learning new information, which could make them vulnerable to the effects of transcultural migration or even rapid changes within the same culture.

Age brings another dimension to the cultural element.

The subculture of older people may bring variations and complexities to the main culture, through their socioeconomic status, gender, or ethnic composition, or different use of language, generational symbols, and cultural interests. Cultures are continually shifting and evolving, sometimes by positive forces but at times by violent conflict or other disruptive forces (Tseng et al., 2004).

Examples of cultural factors in geriatric forensic evaluations

65-year-old East African man is referred for evaluation of competency to stand trial after being charged with assault on a correctional officer. He is a Civil War survivor in his home country. Patient was concerned he was taken away for execution. He had no formal education. He was referred as incompetent and nonrestorable, based primarily on cultural differences. Interpreters were not available. Children tried to help him. Does not understand adversarial nature of the court system.

72-year-old South Korean female widow referred prior to an asylum interview. Argued with her son before leaving her country but the fire in her chest. Stroke killed her husband and son was abusive, and feels pain in her body when she thinks about it.

Holzer et al., 2018

Risk management

Awareness of patient safety, error reduction, and risk management is increasingly important in clinical geriatric psychiatry and in medical-legal applications with the aging of the baby-boomer population and as psychiatric therapeutics gain in complexity.

Regarding patient safety in the geriatric population, there are several important clinical "risk areas" involving elderly patients which can increase the risk of harm. These areas include co-morbid medical illnesses, cognitive dysfunction, and corresponding impaired ability to make informed decisions, sensory input and motor impairments, medication load and side effects, and fall risk. (Holzer et al., 2018).

Adapting techniques from child forensic interviewing

Drawn from decades of research in the field of child abuse, there are several evidence-based protocols used by the forensic interviewers of child advocacy centers who are specially trained and receive ongoing training. Some of these same family dynamics we see are at play when interviewing older adults. For example, older adults may not be forthcoming as they don't want to get their loved one in trouble, and in some of those cases, actually, most of cases, the perpetrator may have actually threatened the older adult, making it even more challenging to get information. To obtain accurate and legally defensible information under some of these difficult circumstances can be pretty challenging. If you look at the research on forensic interviews with older adults, very little has been done to date. The idea of forensic interviewing with older adults has not garnered much attention or funding. But for right now, we definitely need a solution (Gibson, 2017).

Similar family dynamics are often at play in child and elder abuse situations.

Presently, there is no empirically developed curriculum for this type of forensic interviewing with older adults, but hopefully over time that there will be (Gibson, 2017).

Evidence based protocols from child psychiatry

With regards to elder abuse evaluations, the field of child abuse realized this need in the 1980s and began researching how best to elicit accurate information from children, even from very young children. Thirty-five years later, there are several evidence-based protocols used by child advocacy centers' forensic interviewers who are specially trained and receive ongoing training.

- NCAC Child Forensic Interview Structure
- Child First (Finding Words) Training
- Comerhouse Forensic Interview Protocol™
- The NICHD Protocol

Gibson, 2017

Until now, forensic interviewing with older adults has not garnered much attention.

Adapting techniques from child forensic interviewing to older adults

- Not equating children and older adults
- Apply child forensic interviewing principles
- Rapport building
- Open-ended questions

In geriatric forensic evaluations, we definitely need the research to back up our practice.

Medicare billing, documentation and coding

The healthcare industry has placed a great deal of emphasis on documentation requirements, proper coding, and correct billing for services rendered. Practitioners need to understand what is required in documentation of a geriatric psychiatry encounter for an office visit, psychotherapy session, or a forensic evaluation for proper reimbursement. Clinicians should understand what defines fraud and abuse in healthcare. Knowledge of Medicare billing and coding is central to a geriatric psychiatry practice. The CPT code used must be justified in the documentation. (Holzer et al., 2018).

Issues related to Medicare billing and coding are critical to a geriatric psychiatry practice.

Psychopharmacology, black box issues

Prescription drug use is higher among older adults than younger adults. Among people older than 65 years of age, 90% use at least one drug per week, less than 40% use at least five different drugs per week, and 12% use 10 or more drugs per week. Prevalence is especially higher among women, hospitalized patients, and nursing home residents. Elderly patients also experience more drug-related adverse side effects than other age groups.

According to one large study involving ambulatory Medicare patients, 38% of adverse drug events were serious, life-threatening, or fatal; 28% were considered preventable.

Elderly patients experience more drug-related adverse side effects than other age groups.

Atypical antipsychotics are less likely to cause secondary Parkinsonism, although they are not completely devoid of this side-effect. 9 Several studies led the FDA to issue a warning in 2005, stating that use of conventional and atypical antipsychotic drugs to treat dementia-related psychosis in the elderly is associated with an increased risk of death. This risk may be as high as 2.0 times that of placebo. 17 The warning further states that these drugs are not approved for treatment of dementia-related psychosis (Holzer et al., 2018).

Psychiatric home care and telemental health

With the advent of hospitals and improved outpatient care, however, treatment shifted to post-acute care and episodic care, with services including nursing, rehabilitation, and social work. Psychiatric home care and telemental health are two forms of mental health care delivery to homebound mentally ill elderly persons that have the potential to address a wide treatment gap.

Home psychiatric treatment may be considered the preferred modality of addressing the mental health needs of homebound elders, in particular individuals who are cognitively impaired. Telemental health may be able to address the shortage of providers and the cost of home visits. However, telemental health introduces evolving ethical and forensic issues, beyond those encountered in the home visit that clinicians may encounter. (Holzer et al., 2018).

Telemental health introduces evolving ethical and forensic issues.

Long term care issues

Dementia (major neurocognitive disorder), depression, and anxiety disorders are the most prevalent psychiatric disorders among older adults in long-term care. A broad variety of medical-legal issues may arise in the context of identifying psychiatric needs and providing psychiatric care for older persons on a long-term basis. Specific medical-legal and regulatory issues that apply to residents of nursing facilities and assisted living facilities are not encountered in the home and community-based environment. Although the societal and legal deinstitutionalization movement of the last several decades have enabled many extremely disabled older individuals to live in relatively less intrusive home and community-based environments, many geriatric mentally impaired individuals, especially those without sufficient available family support systems, still need to reside and receive care in nursing facilities or assisted living facilities (Holzer et al., 2018).

Suicide

Suicide was the 10th leading cause of death in the United States and the 17th leading cause of death for individuals over the age of 65 in 2013. Suicide risk assessment of older individuals poses a major challenge for healthcare providers.

Suicide risk assessment of older individuals poses a major challenge.

As elderly patients have the highest risk of suicide, clinicians need to be vigilant and implement good clinical practice standards to reduce liability. It is important to be familiar with both general professional guidelines and the risk and protective factors that pertain to their patient's specific situation. Screening tools may help identify suicide risk and track it over time, but they have not been proven to decrease suicidal ideations and suicide. 57 However, screening tools do provide a quantitative measure, and self-reports may facilitate expression by patients who have difficulty disclosing suicide thoughts. Given that suicidality is on a continuum, stratifying the risk severity and temporality in relation to risk factors may assist in ascertaining the actual risk and facilitate clinical decision-making (Holzer et al., 2018).

Consumer protection

Seniors face complex legal concerns that are often different from what they faced when they were younger. A range of federal protections and laws exist offering guidance and regulatory structure to the aging population. Examples reviewed in this chapter include federally supported financial assistance for healthcare and benefits, elder abuse reporting and interventions, consumer protections, and decision-making for the aging and incapacitated. Elder law attorneys focus their practice on the legal needs of seniors and work with a variety of legal tools and techniques to specifically meet the goals of the older client, in order to maximize their autonomy and quality of life (Holzer et al., 2018).

Restoration of rights in guardianship

Adult guardianship has been characterized as both a "gulag and a godsend" in which people with disabilities — including older individuals with dementia — lose their rights in the name of protection. Regardless of the good intentions of — and essential care provided by — many guardians who often step in at crisis points, guardianship is one of society's most drastic interventions in which fundamental rights are transferred to a surrogate, leaving an individual without choice and self-determination.

It appears that an unknown number of adults languish under guardianship beyond the period of need — and that others may never have needed the guardianship in the first place, as a less restrictive option could have sufficed.

When can a guardianship be terminated by the court?

A guardianship may be terminated by the court in these three scenarios:

- If the court finds that the person has regained the ability to make decisions;
- If the court finds that the person has developed sufficient decision-making supports and no longer needs the assistance of a guardian; or
- If additional evidence becomes available to show that the person does not meet the legal standard of an incapacitated person. While, on paper, each state provides for "termination of the order and restoration of rights," there are no data on the frequency with which restoration occurs and under what circumstances.

Wood, 2017

Elder courts

Elder abuse cases are often time consuming and complex, requiring interagency cooperation from a diverse array of professionals. Although multidisciplinary teams (MDTs) offer a potentially powerful approach to synergizing the efforts of different providers, there has been little research on elder abuse MDTs in general or elder abuse forensic centers in particular (Navarro et al., 2010).

The American court system has developed a tradition of specialized court for populations with unique needs. Only a few courts specifically addressing this population are currently set up the US today. It requires close collaboration between legislators, courts and the legal community. Ideally, all parties will work synergistically toward the creation of elder courts (Mintzer, Steinberg et al.)

Conservatorship may be a necessary last resort to improve safety for some FE victims, and the Forensic Center appears to provide a pathway to this service. These findings suggest modification to the Elder Abuse Forensic Center conceptual model and contribute to an emerging body of evidence on the role of the Forensic Center in addressing elder abuse (Gassoumis et al., 2015).

Elder abuse forensic centers present a new model of multidisciplinary collaboration on elder abuse cases. The "clients" of a forensic center are Adult Protective Services (APS), law enforcement, and the Long-term Care Ombudsman. Centers take the basic multidisciplinary team model and add a geriatrician and a psychologist. Additionally, forensic center team members make home visits with APS and others for the purposes of conducting psychological or medical evaluations, lessening the burden of multiple interviews for the alleged abuse victims, and gathering evidence for possible prosecution (Schneider et al., 2010).

Collaboration with elder law attorneys

There are many situations in which an older person needs the services of both an attorney and a physician and communication and collaboration between members of those two professions would be highly advantageous to the older patient/client's well-being. Unfortunately, the record thus far of interprofessional collaboration on behalf of the shared older patient/client in such circumstances generally is deficient and needs to be improved. The first step in the direction of remedying this deficiency must be recognition by both elder law attorneys and physicians (and other health care professionals) of situations in which positive engagement with each other would be valuable for everyone concerned (Kapp et al., 2016).

Topics of collaboration with elder law attorneys:

- Decisional capacity
- Elder mistreatment
- Self-neglect
- Medical payment
- Family issues
- Confidentiality

Kapp et al., 2016

Lawyers with clients who have diminished capacity play an important role in protecting the interests of the vulnerable in society. Increasingly those engaged in working with clients who are mentally ill, elderly, or experiencing fluctuating mental capacity, are called upon to make decisions and protect interests of clients who struggle to understand the legal consequence and meaning of their decisions. Ethical principles that prohibit lawyers from acting on anything other than (legally) competent instructions, and that disapprove of acting 'in the best interests' of clients in the absence of competent instructions, creates a series of philosophical and practical challenges to lawyers who work in this area (Castles, 2015).

Residency and fellowship training

The number of older persons involved with the legal system has increased because this age group's population has increased and due to elder-related issues, such as conflicts over inheritance, disputes regarding healthcare and other care and management issues, and elder abuse, coming before the courts. In addition, in many jurisdictions, lengthy prison sentences have resulted in an aging prison population. Forensic assessments of the elderly will therefore be called for more frequently, most often involving questions of capacity due to the increased frequency of neurocognitive impairment with aging. To have expertise in geriatric forensic psychiatry, clearly one needs training in both forensics and geriatrics, a double fellowship qualification held by very few psychiatrists.

Double fellowship qualification in both forensics and geriatrics is held by very few psychiatrists.

Opportunities exist to adapt training within existing fellowships, with the goal of providing the services that courts will require in order to best protect the interests and rights of the aging population. The current Accreditation Council for Graduate Medical Education (ACGME) requirements for forensic psychiatry and geriatric psychiatry fellowship training are fundamental to ensure that these curricula will provide optimal experiences to prepare graduates for this subtle and complex work. Other issues that need to be addressed include considerations for training in forensic geriatric issues in medical education, training for non-physician healthcare providers, and addressing future policy to ensure the availability of persons who will be needed for this growing area of forensic activity (Holzer et al., 2018).

Current ACGME requirements for ethics/legal in geriatric psychiatry fellowship:

- Competence
- Capacity
- Guardianship
- Right to refuse treatment
- Wills
- Advance directives
- Informed consent
- Elder abuse
- Withholding of medical treatments
- Federal legislative guidelines governing psychotropic drug prescription in nursing homes and other settings

Holzer et al., 2018

ABPN proposed forensic psychiatry core competencies relevant to geriatric issues:

- Assessment of competence
- Guardianship
- Advance directives
- Right to refuse treatment
- Wills
- Informed consent
- Elder abuse
- Withholding of medical treatment
- End-of-life issues
- Palliative care
- Federal legislative guidelines governing psychotropic medication prescribing in nursing

Holzer et al., 2018

Future needs

Going forward, there are many future needs to improve geriatric forensic evaluations, including:

- specific measures of decision-making capacities across normal aging, long term impairment, and Alzheimer's disease
- instruments that help measure and prevent financial exploitation and unintentional self-impoverishment by older adults making poor decisions over time
- awareness, time, and reimbursement for physicians and other clinicians to do this work
- implementation of streamlined and standardized instruments
- multidisciplinary teamwork and seamless coordination among all interested parties

Conclusion

As practicing clinicians caring for elderly patients, we are increasingly faced with questions about decision-making capacity and other medicolegal issues. We clinicians can work together with other members of a multidisciplinary team to improve forensic evaluations in older adults. Though geriatric forensic evaluations are often challenging, it can be interpersonally meaningful and professionally rewarding for clinicians to implement competent skills in this area.

Selected references

ABA/APA Working Group, 2008. Judicial Determination of Capacity of Older Adults: A Handbook for Judges.

American Bar Association Commission on Law and Aging, C. o. D. R., Section on Civil Rights and Social Justice; and Section on Real Property, Trust and Estate Law, 2016. Practical Tool for Lawyers: Steps in Supporting Decision-Making.

Blanck, P., Martinis, J.G., 2015. "The right to make choices": the national resource center for supported decision-making. Inclusion 3 (1), 24–33.

Castles, M., 2015. Mind the gaps: ethical representation of clients with questionable mental capacity. Leg. Ethics 18 (1), 24–45.

Gassoumis, Z.D., Navarro, A.E., Wilber, K.H., 2015. Protecting victims of elder financial exploitation: the role of an Elder Abuse Forensic Center in referring victims for conservatorship. Aging Ment. Health 19 (9), 790–798.

Gibson, S., 2017. Forensic Interviewing with Older Adults. U.S. Department of Justice, Elder Justice Initiative. https://www.justice.gov/elderjustice/video/forensic-interviewing-older-adults.

Hess, T.M., Strough, J.N., Löckenhoff, C., 2015. Aging and Decision Making: Empirical and Applied Perspectives. Elsevier Science.
Holzer, J.C., Kohn, R., Ellison, M., Recupero, P.R., 2018. Geriatric forensic psychiatry: principles and practice. Oxford University Press, New York, NY.
Justice, U. S. D. o., 2018. Elder Justice Initiative (EJI): Financial Exploitation Website from. https://www.justice.gov/elderjustice/financial-exploitation.
Kapp, M.B., 2010. Older clients with questionable legal competence: elder law practitioners and treating physicians. Wm. Mitchell L. Rev. 37, 99.
Kapp, M.B., Taite, S.M., Turner, G., 2016. Six situations in which elder law attorneys and physicians caring for older patients need each other. Bifocal 37 (6), 115–118.
Mintzer, J., E. S. Steinberg and J. L. Pearson "Elder courts: a new way to protect the frail elderly population." Am. J. Geriatr. Psychiatry 23(3): S31.
Navarro, A.E., Wilber, K.H., Yonashiro, J., Homeier, D.C., 2010. Do we really need another meeting? Lessons from the Los Angeles county elder abuse forensic center. Gerontol. 50 (5), 702–711.
Peck, K., Law, R.L., Peck, B., Law, D., American Bar Association, Senior Lawyers Division, 2013. Alzheimer's and the Law: Counseling Clients with Dementia and Their Families. ABA, Senior Lawyers Division, Chicago, Illinois.
Plotkin, D.A., Spar, J.E., Horwitz, H.L., 2016. "Assessing Undue Influence." J Am Acad Psychiatry Law 44 (3), 344–351.
Roesch, R., Zapf, P.A., 2013. Forensic Assessments in Criminal and Civil Law: A Handbook for Lawyers. Oxford University Press, New York.
R. L. Sadoff. Future Directions. New York, Oxford University Press: 155-162.
Schneider, D.C., Mosqueda, L., Falk, E., Huba, G.J., 2010. Elder abuse forensic centers. J. Elder Abuse Negl. 22 (3–4), 255–274.
Silva, J.A., 2009. Forensic psychiatry, neuroscience, and the law. J Am. Acad. Psychiat. Law 37 (4), 489.
Stakeholders, W. W. I. N. o. G., 2018. WINGS – Stakeholder Networks for Guardianship Reform from. https://ambar.org/wings.
Streim, J.E., 2015. Forensic Issues in Geriatric Psychiatry. The Evolution of Forensic Psychiatry: History, Current Developments.
Tampi, R.R., Young, J., Balachandran, S., Dasarathy, D., Tampi, D., 2018. Ethical, legal and forensic issues in geriatric psychiatry. Curr. Psychiatr. Rep. 20 (1), 1.
Taylor, M.H., Grossberg, G.T., 2012. The growing problem of illicit substance abuse in the elderly: a review. Prim. Care Companion CNS Disord. 14 (4).
Tseng, W.-S., Matthews, D.B., Elwyn, T.S., 2004. Cultural Competence in Forensic Mental Health: A Guide for Psychiatrists, Psychologists, and Attorneys. Brunner-Routledge, New York.
U. S. Senate, 2016. Trust Betrayed: Financial Abuse of Older Americans by Guardians and Others in Power.
ULC, 2017. UAGPPJA – Uniform Adult Guardianship and Protective Proceedings Act.
ULC, 2017. UGCOPPA – Uniform Guardianship, Conservatorship and Other Protective Arrangements Act.
Wald, M., Pierce, E.D., 2016. Elder ethics: how supported decision-making could protect incapacitated seniors. TEX. B. J. 79, 104.
website, N. R. C. f. S. D. M, 2018. National Resource Center for Supported Decision Making.
Wood, E., 2016. Recharging Adult Guardianship Reform.
Wood, E., 2017. Restoration of Rights in Adult Guardianship: Research and Recommendations.

Woods, A.J., Porges, E.C., Bryant, V.E., Seider, T., Gongvatana, A., Kahler, C.W., de la Monte, S., Monti, P.M., Cohen, R.A., 2016. Current heavy alcohol consumption is associated with greater cognitive impairment in older adults. Alcohol Clin. Exp. Res. 40 (11), 2435–2444.

Woods, B., Pratt, R., 2005. Awareness in dementia: ethical and legal issues in relation to people with dementia. Aging Ment. Health 9 (5), 423–429.

Yarnell, S.C., Kirwin, P.D., Zonana, H.V., 2017. Geriatrics and the legal system. J Am. Acad. Psychiat. Law 45 (2), 208.

Sample psychiatric report

Executive summary

This is an expert Psychiatric Report in the matter of Carolyn Jones – Will Contest, Case 0000–0001, submitted to Marvin Smith, Attorney, by Karen Reimers, MD, Psychiatrist.

Mrs. Carolyn Jones signed a will on August 8, 2014 at 95 years of age while living in residential care at Cumberland Care Center in Cumberland, Maine. Mrs. Jones' 2014 will replaced her 1999 will, which she had signed when she was 80 years old, prior to the death of her husband William Jones Sr. in 2000.

Mrs. Jones' son Alexander Jones and daughter Caitlyn Matthews are co-executors of her 2014 will, which leaves the bulk of her estate to them, her surviving children. Mrs. Jones' grandsons Todd Jones and Brian Jones, sons of Mrs. Jones' deceased son William Jones Jr., who died in 2009, are the plaintiffs in the current will contest case.

Based on review of available records, my education, training and experience, it is my expert psychiatric opinion that four problems interfered with Mrs. Jones' ability to make her will in 2014: dementia, medical illness and physical frailty, polypharmacy (multiple medications), and emotional vulnerability.

For these reasons, Mrs. Jones did not have the mental ability to make a will in August 2014.

Mrs. Jones was susceptible to undue influence at the time her 2014 will was made, due to her frail physical, mental and emotional state.

Background

This is the will contest of Mrs. Carolyn Jones' 2014 will,[1] which she signed on August 8, 2014 at 95 years of age while living in residential care at Cumberland Care Center in Cumberland, Maine. Mrs. Jones' 2014 will

[1] Exhibit 3, Deposition Exhibits 1–19, 3/17/2017.

replaced her 1999 will,[2] which she signed when she was 80 years old, prior to the death of her husband William Sr. in 2000. Over the years, Mrs. Jones made statements that she had wanted to keep her 1999 will in place.[3]

Mrs. Jones' son Alexander Jones and daughter Caitlyn Matthews are co-executors of her 2014 will, which leaves the bulk of the family estate to them, her surviving children. Mrs. Jones' 2014 will does not reference that Mrs. Jones had only an undivided one-half interest in the real estate.[4] Mrs. Jones' grandsons Todd Jones and Brian Jones, sons of Mrs. Jones' son William Jones Jr. who died in 2009, are plaintiffs in the current will contest. Their mother Marlene Jones, widow of Mrs. Jones' son William Jones Jr., also provided deposition testimony in this case.

Key events in Mrs. Jones' life

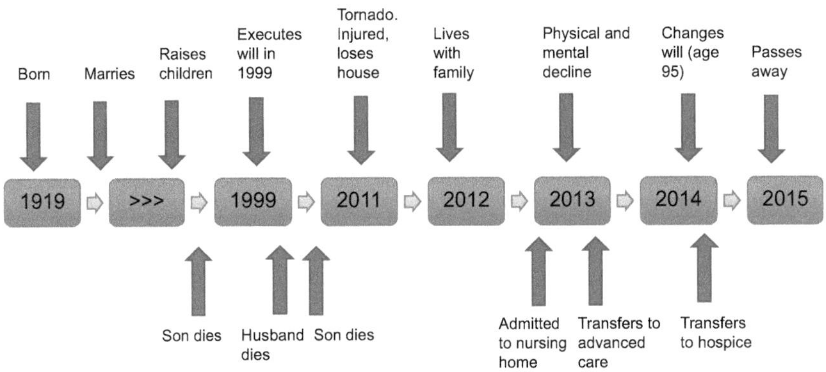

Born in 1919, Mrs. Jones spent most of her life as a farm wife in Cumberland County, Maine. She and her husband William Jones Sr. raised 4 children, including three sons, Richard Jones, William Jones Jr., Alexander Jones and one daughter Caitlyn Matthews (Roman). Unfortunately, her son Richard Jones was killed in an accident in the 1990s, and her son William Jones Jr. died in 2009 after a lengthy illness.

[2] Exhibit 2, Deposition Exhibits 1–19, 3/17/2017.

[3] Deposition of Timothy Jones (Plaintiff), 3/17/2017, p. 63; Deposition of Marlene Jones (Mother of Plaintiffs and daughter-in-law of Decedent, Carolyn Jones), 3/17/2017, p. 27–28; Deposition of Brian Jones (Plaintiff), 3/17/2017, p. 33; Answers to Interrogatories which were executed and served by plaintiffs, 12/7/2016, p. 14.

[4] Answers to Interrogatories which were executed and served by plaintiffs, 12/7/2016, p. 14.

Following the death of Mrs. Jones' husband William Sr. in 2000, most of the family's property was converted to a lifetime trust in Mrs. Jones' name, to be owned and managed by Mrs. Jones until her death. Mrs. Jones' son Alexander Jones managed the financial aspects of the farm business with Mrs. Jones' permission. Alexander Jones signed checks on Mrs. Jones' bank accounts.[5] Alexander Jones leased out part of the family land and collected rent, consulting with tax professionals to prepare his and Mrs. Jones' tax returns. In 2014, Alexander Jones provided Mrs. Jones with a modest annual allowance of $26,000, while keeping a much larger amount from the farm's proceeds for himself.[6] Mrs. Jones was concerned about Alexander's financial situation and debts,[7] and allowed him to keep a sizable proportion of proceeds from the family farm.

Mrs. Jones suffered from chronic anxiety and depression, as well as progressively worsening memory problems. She was treated with numerous psychiatric medications over the years. She suffered from chronic pain and multiple medical problems.

Tornado

A tornado in April 2011 left Mrs. Jones injured and destroyed her house, where she had previously been living independently. Mrs. Jones was hospitalized at Cumberland Medical Center in April 2011 and then lived with her children temporarily until being admitted to Cumberland Ridgeview Care Center in Cumberland, Maine in January 2013. She transferred to Cumberland Care Center in Cumberland, Maine in October 2013. Throughout this time and for the rest of her final years she was physically frail, unable to care for herself, walk without assistance or use the bathroom independently. Records indicate she also developed significant memory problems consistent with moderate dementia starting in or before 2013.[8]

5 Deposition of Alexander Jones (Co-Executor), 3/17/2017, p. 58.

6 Exhibit 22, Deposition Exhibits 20–42, 3/17/2017; Deposition of Timothy Jones (Plaintiff), 3/17/2017, p. 51.

7 Deposition of Timothy Jones (Plaintiff), 3/17/2016, p. 49.

8 Universal Health medical records (Bates stamped 748–832), 2011–4, p. 24, p. 21, p. 32, p. 36; Cumberland Hospital medical records (Bates stamped 123–747), 2011–4, p. 134; Answers to Interrogatories which were executed and served by plaintiffs, 12/7/2016, 12/7/2016, p. 11; Deposition of Brian Jones (Plaintiff), 3/17/2017, p. 25.

New will

On August 7, 2014, an attorney, Alexander Jones and Caitlyn Matthews meet with Mrs. Jones at Cumberland Care Center nursing home to discuss making a new will. Since Mrs. Jones was too frail to go to the attorney's office, Alexander Jones had arranged for the attorney to go to her room at the nursing home. The attorney's handwritten notes from their group discussion on August 7, 2014 indicate splitting 400 acres equally into 200 acres each for Alexander Jones and Caitlyn Matthews respectively.[9] After the meeting, the lawyer prepared documents. Alexander Jones went to the attorney's office to pick up the prepared documents and bring them to his mother in the nursing home the next day.[10]

Signing the new will

On August 8, 2014, at 95 years of age, Mrs. Jones signed a last will and testament, with her son Alexander Jones and daughter Caitlyn Matthews as co-executors.[11] The attorney was not present at the meeting on August 8, 2014 when the will was signed. With Alexander Jones and Caitlyn Matthews in her room, lying in her bed, Mrs. Jones signed the 2014 will document. The nursing home administrator acted as notary and 2 staff from the nursing home served as witnesses.[12] That day, Mrs. Jones complained of not feeling well.[13]

Mrs. Jones' physical and mental health continued to decline. Her condition deteriorated considerably in August 2014 and beyond, with multiple medication changes, falls, progressive dementia, and a stroke shortly before her death.[14] Mrs. Jones transferred to East River Care Center in East River, Maine in October 2014. Mrs. Jones died at East River Care Center on April 10, 2015, eight months after signing her 2014 will.

Following her death, Mrs. Jones' 2014 will was admitted to probate with Cumberland County. The first notice of probate of the will was published on May 12, 2015 and the second notice of probate of the will was published on

[9] Exhibit 40, Deposition Exhibits 20–42, 3/17/2017.

[10] Deposition of Caitlyn Matthews/Roman (Co-Executor), 3/17/2017, p. 30.

[11] Exbibit 3, Deposition Exhibits 1–19, 3/17/2017.

[12] Deposition of Caitlyn Matthews/Roman (Co-Executor), 3/17/2017, p. 28.

[13] Cumberland Care Center nursing home records (Bates stamped 1390–2143), 2013–4, p. 179.

[14] Cumberland Care Center nursing home records (Bates stamped 1390–2143), 2013–4, p. 24, 78, 107, 111, 140, 150, 166; Cumberland Hospital medical records (Bates stamped 123–747), 2011–4, p. 538, 539, 559; East River Care Center nursing home records (Bates stamped 834–1389), 2014–5, p. 18.

May 27, 2015. Petition to set aside/contest probate of will was filed in August 2015 by plaintiffs Tim and Brian Jones, grandsons of Mrs. Jones, against Caitlyn Matthews and Alexander Jones, co-executors of the estate of Mrs. Jones.

Questions to address

1. Did Mrs. Jones have the mental ability to make a will in August 2014?
2. Was Mrs. Jones susceptible to undue influence in August 2014?

Qualifications

I am a Medical Doctor with specialization and board certification in Psychiatry. My professional activities include clinical work treating patients, teaching at two local training programs for Psychiatry residents, and research. In my clinical practice, I care for adult patients including elderly patients with dementia and complex medical problems.

I received my M.D. degree from the Ludwig Maximilian University of Munich in 2008, and a BA degree from McGill University in 2000. I am a Board Certified in Psychiatry by American Academy of Psychiatry and Neurology. I am licensed to practice medicine in Minnesota and Wisconsin. I am active in several professional associations including the American Psychiatric Association, the American Association for Geriatric Psychiatry, the American Academy of Psychosomatic Medicine, and American Academy for Psychiatry and the Law.

I completed four years of residency in Psychiatry at the State University of New York, in Buffalo. I worked as a Psychiatrist at Mayo Clinic in Eau Claire, Wisconsin from 2013 until 2016. Since then, I have been practicing adult Psychiatry in the greater Twin Cities area and rural Wisconsin.

The following list includes selected projects relevant to this case:

- Adjunct Assistant Professor at University of Minnesota, Department of Psychiatry
- Designed, developed and taught lectures for Psychiatry residents on Geriatric Psychiatry, Psychosomatic Medicine, and Forensic Psychiatry at the University of Minnesota and the Regions-Hennepin training programs, 2016–7

- Lectured on Driving Capacity in the Elderly at American Association of Geriatric Psychiatry Annual Meeting, Dallas, 2017
- Lectured on Geriatric Forensic Evaluations at the Annual Meeting of the Midwest Chapter, American Academy for Psychiatry and the Law, Kansas City, 2017
- Lectured and facilitated psychiatric case reviews with Family Medicine residents and faculty at University of Wisconsin Family Medicine residency training program, Eau Claire, Wisconsin, 2014–5
- Published peer-reviewed article "Capgras-like visual hallucinations in Lewy Body Dementia with therapeutic response to donepezil" in Neurology Clinical Practice (2013)
- Fellow of American Psychiatric Association
- Member of multiple committees at American Association for Geriatric Psychiatry and American Academy for Psychiatry and the Law
- Board-certified Fellow of the Royal College of Physicians of Canada, member of Canadian Psychiatric Association and Canadian Association for Geriatric Psychiatry

My resume is attached for reference.

Documents reviewed

I consulted, reviewed, and analyzed the following documents in the preparation of this report:

1. Petition to Set Aside Will, 8/20/2015
2. Ridgeview Care Center nursing home records (Bates stamped 1–122), 2013
3. Cumberland Hospital medical records (Bates stamped 123–747), 2011–4
4. Universal Health medical records (Bates stamped 748–832), 2011–4
5. East River Care Center nursing home records (Bates stamped 834–1389), 2014–5
6. Cumberland Care Center nursing home records (Bates stamped 1390–2143), 2013–4
7. Answers to Interrogatories which were executed and served by plaintiffs, 12/7/2016
8. Deposition of Alexander Jones (Co-Executor), 3/17/2017
9. Deposition of Caitlyn Matthews/Roman (Co-Executor), 3/17/2017

10. Deposition of Timothy Jones (Plaintiff), 3/17/2017
11. Deposition of Brian Jones (Plaintiff), 3/17/2017
12. Deposition of Marlene Jones (Mother of Plaintiffs and daughter-in-law of Decedent, Carolyn Jones), 3/17/2017
13. Deposition Exhibits 1–19, 3/17/2017
14. Deposition Exhibits 20–42, 3/17/2017
15. Deposition Exhibits 101 & 102, 3/17/2017

I also reviewed the following references from the literature:

1. American Geriatrics Society 2015 Beers Criteria Update Expert Panel (2015). American Geriatrics Society 2015 Updated Beers Criteria for Potentially Inappropriate Medication Use in Older Adults. J Am Geriatr Soc 63:2227–2246.
2. American Psychiatric Association (2013). Diagnostic and statistical manual of mental disorders: DSM-5. Arlington, VA, American Psychiatric Association.
3. Centers for Medicare and Medicaid Services (2016). Long-Term Care Facility Resident Assessment 3.0 User's Manual, Version 1.14. United States Department of Health and Human Services. Available at https://downloads.cms.gov/files/MDS-30-RAI-Manual-V114-October-2016.pdf
4. Chen, X. et al. (2014). Frailty syndrome: an overview. Clinical Interventions in Aging (2014):9 433–441.
5. Chodosh, J. et al. (2008). Nursing Home Assessment of Cognitive Impairment: Development and Testing of a Brief Instrument of Mental Status. J Am Geriatr Soc 56:2069–75.
6. Mart, E. G. and AD. Alban (2011). The practical assessment of testamentary capacity and undue influence in the elderly. Sarasota, Florida, Professional Resource Press.
7. Olfson, M. et al. (2015). Benzodiazepine Use in the United States. JAMA Psychiatry 72(2):136–142.
8. Peisah, C., J. Luxenberg, B. Liptzin, A. P. Wand, K. Shulman and S. Finkel (2014). Deathbed wills: assessing testamentary capacity in the dying patient. Int Psychogeriatr 26(2): 209–216.
9. Shaik, S. et al. (2012). Differentiating the dementias: a neurological approach. Progress in Neurology and Psychiatry 16(1):11–18.
10. Shulman, K. I., C. A. Cohen and I. Hull (2005). Psychiatric issues in retrospective challenges of testamentary capacity. International Journal of Geriatric Psychiatry 20(1): 63–69.

11. Shulman, K. I., C. A. Cohen, F. C. Kirsh, I. M. Hull and P. R. Champine (2007). Assessment of testamentary capacity and vulnerability to undue influence. American Journal of Psychiatry 164(5): 722–727.
12. Spar, J. E. and A. S. Garb (1992). Assessing competency to make a will. American Journal of Psychiatry 149(2): 169.

Methodology

At the time of my review of this case, Mrs. Jones was deceased and could not be directly assessed. I conducted a retrospective evaluation of her mental ability to make a will and her susceptibility to undue influence, limiting the basis of my opinions to information available from medical records and other collateral sources: the documents, deposition reports, hospital and nursing home records listed under "Documents Reviewed" above. The records in this case are voluminous. Although I have reviewed all the records provided to me, in this report I focus on evidence that throws light on Mrs. Jones' mental ability to make a will and her ability to resist undue influence.

Findings

Four causes of impaired mental ability to make a will and susceptibility to undue influence

In my expert opinion, based on review of available medical records, the following four problem areas caused impairment of Mrs. Jones' mental ability to make a will and made her susceptible to undue influence:

1. Dementia
2. Medical illness and physical frailty
3. Polypharmacy (multiple medications)
4. Emotional vulnerability

Below I will address the available records that shows how each of these four problems impaired Mrs. Jones' mental capacity to make a will and made her susceptible to undue influence.

Dementia

Dementia (Major Neurocognitive Disorder) describes significant cognitive decline that interferes with everyday activities. Patients with dementia may have problems with complex attention, executive function, learning and memory, language, perceptual and motor function, and/or social cognition.[15] Memory problems are usually prominent in patients with dementia. In Mrs. Jones' case, family members acknowledge that she had significant periods of forgetfulness.[16]

Dementia often begins insidiously. Despite their memory impairment, many patients with dementia who have preserved social graces are preserved seem engaging and conversant, even if they are not able to remember information or answer orientation questions.[17]

Though formal neuropsychological testing was not performed in this case, evidence from available records indicates Mrs. Jones suffered from a progressive dementia that was at least moderate in degree, starting in at least 2013.[18] Mrs. Jones was noted to have forgetfulness and dementia by multiple physicians and other care providers who evaluated her during her lifetime, including Dr. Peters and Dr. Gregory.[19] For example, Dr. Peters' discharge summary from Cumberland Care Center dated October 8, 2014 specifically lists dementia among numerous other medical and psychiatric diagnoses.[20]

Brief Interview of Mental Status (BIMS)

Cognitive assessment is a required component of the federally mandated assessment of nursing home residents in the United States.[21] Beyond being diagnosed with dementia by her treating physicians, Mrs. Jones underwent regular cognitive screening assessments which revealed cognitive deficits that worsened over time, consistent with the typical progressive course of

15 American Psychiatric Association (2013). Diagnostic and statistical manual of mental disorders: DSM-5. Arlington, VA, American Psychiatric Association, p. 591.

16 Deposition of Caitlyn Matthews/Roman (Co-Executor), 3/17/2017, p. 47; Deposition of Marlene Jones (Mother of Plaintiffs and daughter-in-law of Decedent, Carolyn Jones), 3/17/2017, p. 26.

17 Shaik, S. et al. (2012). Differentiating the dementias: a neurological approach. Progress in Neurology and Psychiatry 16(1):11–18, p. 13.

18 Cumberland Hospital medical records (Bates stamped 123–747), 2011–4, p. 134, 136.

19 Universal Health medical records (Bates stamped 748–832), 2011–4, p. 23, 34, 35.

20 Cumberland Care Center nursing home records (Bates stamped 1390–2143), 2013–4, p. 22.

21 Centers for Medicare and Medicaid Services (2016). Long-Term Care Facility Resident Assessment 3.0 User's Manual, Version 1.14. United States Department of Health and Human Services. Available at https://downloads.cms.gov/files/MDS-30-RAI-Manual-V114-October-2016.pdf, p. C1.

dementia. In Mrs. Jones' case, the tool used for this federally mandated cognitive assessment was the Brief Interview of Mental Status (BIMS), which is a brief, simply scored screen for cognitive function.[22] The BIMS assessment consists of 3 parts:

- Repetition of three words
- Orientation to year, month and current day of the week
- Recall of the 3 words from first step

To determine the patient's level of cognitive impairment, the BIMS assigns simple whole numbers to each item, for a total maximum score of 15. Assessment categories for the BIMS are:

- BIMS score of 13–15: little to no impairment
- BIMS score of 8–12: moderate cognitive impairment
- BIMS score of 0–7: severe cognitive impairment

Scores on BIMS indicate progressive cognitive decline

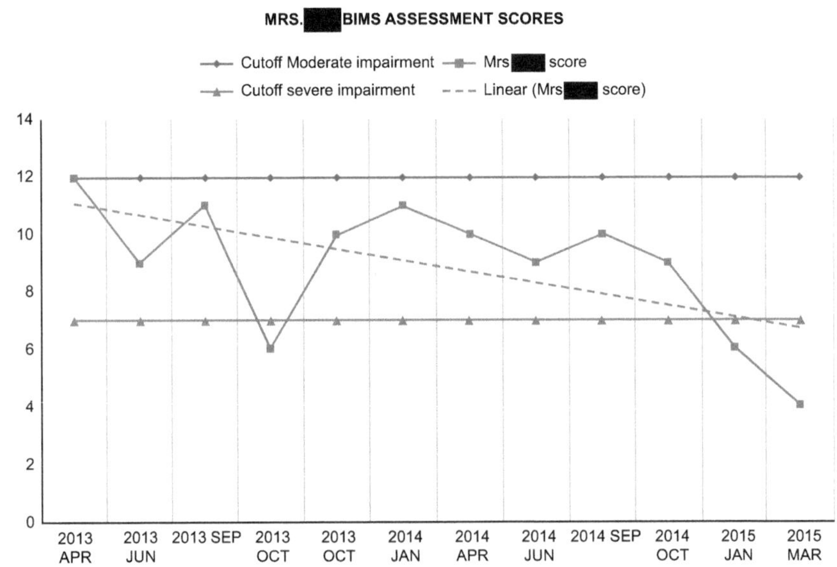

As depicted by the diagram above, Mrs. Jones' scores on the BIMs deteriorated over time, indicating moderate to severe cognitive impairment.

[22] Chodosh, J. et al. (2008). Nursing Home Assessment of Cognitive Impairment: Development and Testing of a Brief Instrument of Mental Status. J Am Geriatr Soc 56:2069–75, p. 2070.

This is a common pattern among dementia patients, consistent with progressive dementia. By the time she signed the will in August 2014, Mrs. Jones' BIMS score was in the moderate range of cognitive impairment. By the time she died 8 months later, Mrs. Jones' BIMS score was in the severe range of cognitive impairment.

Impaired executive function

BIMS assessments are rapid screening tests to assess global cognition, but the BIMS does not assess executive function, a key area of cognitive impairment in dementia. Executive function refers to the ability to control behavior and make complex decisions.

Evidence from the records reveals many documented examples of Mrs. Jones' behavior and statements indicating that she had compromised executive function.[23] Like many patients with dementia, Mrs. Jones had minimal insight into her memory problems.[24] Mrs. Jones had problems with judgment and impulse control; for example, she would impulsively get up and try to walk to the bathroom without assistance, leading to numerous falls, and at times she would repeatedly ring the nurse call alarm unnecessarily.[25] Mrs. Jones had difficulty with organization and planning.[26] Though evidence from the records suggests Mrs. Jones' social graces remained mostly intact, she occasionally demonstrated problems with empathy, a sign of executive dysfunction. For example, Mrs. Jones at times verbalize paranoid or hurtful comments to nursing home staff.[27] Such outbursts are inconsistent with her baseline demeanor and are most likely explained by progressive dementia. Mrs. Jones had major problems with motivation. In her final years, records indicate she was generally uninterested in new activities, appeared apathetic, and needed direction or assistance from others to engage in almost any activity.[28] Mrs. Jones refused to get out of bed, at times even

23 East River Care Center nursing home records (Bates stamped 834—1389), 2014—5; Cumberland Care Center nursing home records (Bates stamped 1390—2143), 2013—4.

24 Cumberland Care Center nursing home records (Bates stamped 1390—2143), 2013—4, p. 67.

25 Cumberland Care Center nursing home records (Bates stamped 1390—2143), 2013—4, p. 177, 244.

26 Ridgeview Care Center nursing home records (Bates stamped 1—122), 2013, p. 3, 5, 10, 117, 119, 122. Cumberland Care Center nursing home records (Bates stamped 1390—2143), 2013—4, p. 132, 182, 220.

27 Ridgeview Care Center nursing home records (Bates stamped 1—122), 2013, p. 120. Cumberland Care Center nursing home records (Bates stamped 1390—2143), 2013—4, p. 168, 206. East River Care Center nursing home records (Bates stamped 834—1389), 2014—5, p. 29, 44, 515, 530.

28 Ridgeview Care Center nursing home records (Bates stamped 1—122), 2013, p. 122. East River Care Center nursing home records (Bates stamped 834—1389), 2014—5, p. 209.

refused to bathe for long stretches time, uncharacteristic of her behavior prior to dementia.[29] Apathy and the behavior patterns described here are commonly seen in dementia patients. In Mrs. Jones' case, the evidence indicates that her apathy and problematic behaviors were very likely due to her advancing dementia.

Mrs. Jones appears to have enjoyed reading throughout her life. In her final years, Mrs. Jones spent her days in bed, and reading was one of the few activities she could engage in. Reading was a socially appropriate activity for Mrs. Jones that was encouraged by staff and family, who brought her books and newspapers. No formal neuropsychological testing was done to assess Mrs. Jones' reading comprehension level, but given her cognitive impairments including short term memory loss, in her final years Mrs. Jones would have had great difficulty with reading. Despite the superficial appearance of Mrs. Jones reading various documents in her final years, is unlikely she understood the content of what she was reading.[30] A few months before her death, when her cognition was moderately to severely impaired, a nurse practitioner at East River Care Center noted that Mrs. Jones continued to act as if she was reading the newspaper, even as the nurse practitioner performed a physical exam.[31] Such inflexible, stereotyped behavior would have been uncharacteristic of Mrs. Jones prior to her cognitive impairment, but it is relatively common in individuals with advanced dementia.

Medical illness and frailty

At the time Mrs. Jones signed her 2014 will, she suffered from numerous medical problems. Her treating physician Dr. Peters compiled a list of 26 of Mrs. Jones' most important medical problems on October 8, 2014, for the discharge summary at the time of transfer from Cumberland Care Center to East River Care Center.[32]

Mrs. Jones' 26 diagnoses are listed here in alphabetical order. Except for the right foot fracture she sustained on August 22, 2014, Mrs. Jones' 26 diagnoses listed by Dr. Peters were all active and relevant at the time of the signing of the will on August 8, 2014. In addition to these 26 diagnoses, other records indicate further prior medical diagnoses for Mrs. Jones, including a history of transient ischemic attacks (mini strokes) in the early 1990s.[33]

[29] Cumberland Care Center nursing home records (Bates stamped 1390—2143), 2013—4, p. 177, 210.
[30] Cumberland Care Center nursing home records (Bates stamped 1390—2143), 2013—4, p. 166.
[31] East River Care Center nursing home records (Bates stamped 834—1389), 2014—5, p. 209.
[32] Cumberland Care Center nursing home records (Bates stamped 1390—2143), 2013—4, p. 21—26.
[33] Cumberland Hospital medical records (Bates stamped 123—747), 2011—4, p. 105.

Mrs. Jones' 26 medical diagnoses

1. Anxiety state
2. Atherosclerosis of renal artery
3. Atrial fibrillation
4. Cardiac arrhythmia
5. Dementia
6. Depression
7. Dysthymic disorder
8. Essential hypertension
9. Foot fracture (sustained August 22, 2014)
10. Generalized osteoarthritis involving multiple sites
11. Hereditary and idiopathic peripheral neuropathy
12. Hyperlipidemia
13. Hypocalcemia
14. Impaired fasting glucose
15. Lumbago
16. Mixed and stress incontinence
17. Occlusion and stenosis of carotid artery
18. Osteoporosis
19. Other malaise and fatigue
20. Pain in thoracic spine
21. Psychosis
22. Sciatica
23. Thoracic or lumbosacral neuritis or radiculitis
24. Unspecified constipation
25. Unspecified hypothyroidism
26. Vitamin D deficiency

Due to her multiple impairments, Mrs. Jones could not cope adequately with everyday stresses. She was completely dependent on her caregivers and family for her basic needs, including walking, bathing and going to the bathroom.[34] Clearly, Mrs. Jones struggled with considerable weakness, feebleness and frailty.[35] Mrs. Jones met criteria for frailty syndrome, with its age associated declines in function and increased vulnerability.

[34] Cumberland Care Center nursing home records (Bates stamped 1390–2143), 2013–4, p. 493.

[35] Cumberland Hospital medical records (Bates stamped 123–747), 2011–4, p. 206, 317. Deposition of Alexander Jones (Co-Executor), 3/17/2017, p. 22. Cumberland Care Center nursing home records (Bates stamped 1390–2143), 2013–4, p. 18, 190.

Mrs. Jones met frailty syndrome criteria[36]

- Weakness
- Slowness
- Low level of physical activity
- Self-reported exhaustion
- Unintentional weight loss

Polypharmacy (multiple medications)

Elderly people are sensitive to adverse effects from medications. Polypharmacy (prescription of multiple concurrent medications) is a risk factor for confusion and cognitive impairment. As more medications are prescribed, there is increased potential for harmful drug-drug interactions. Mrs. Jones' treating physicians had the challenging task of prescribing in this complicated context, weighing the various risks and benefits of the numerous treatments needed for her multiple serious medical problems, including chronic anxiety. Below is the list of the 23 medications that were prescribed for Mrs. Jones at Cumberland Care Center on the day she signed her 2014 will, including her 13 scheduled and 10 as-needed medications:

Mrs. Jones' 23 medications[37]

1. Amiodarone 200 mg tablet by mouth daily at noon
2. Amlodipine Besylate 5 mg tablet by mouth twice daily
3. Aspirin 81 mg tablet daily at noon
4. Calcium carbonate-Vitamin D 500-125 mg-unit tablet by mouth daily at 8 a.m.
5. Citalopram Hydrobromide 20 mg tablet by mouth daily at 8 p.m.
6. Clorazepate Dipotassium 7.5 mg tablet by mouth daily at 8 a.m.
7. Docusate Sodium 100 mg capsule by mouth daily at noon
8. Levothyroxine Sodium 100 mcg tablet by mouth daily at 8 a.m.
9. Lorazepam 0.25 mg tablet by mouth twice daily starting 7/29/14, last dose on 8/12/14
10. Naproxen 375 mg tablet by mouth every bedtime
11. Omeprazole delayed release 20 mg capsule once daily at 8 a.m.

36 Chen, X. et al. (2014). Frailty syndrome: an overview. Clinical Interventions in Aging (2014):9 433–441, p. 434.

37 Cumberland Care Center nursing home records (Bates stamped 1390–2143), 2013–4, p. 429–456.

12. Polyethylene Glycol 3350 17 gm powder by mouth in juice daily at 8 a.m.
13. Vitamin D3 5000-unit capsule by mouth three times weekly
14. Acetaminophen 500 mg 1 to 2 tablets by mouth every 6 h as needed for pain (1000 mg dose given twice daily on both 8/7/14 and 8/8/14)
15. Artificial tears 1.4% Ophthalmic solution 1 drop into both eyes four times daily as needed for dry eyes
16. Aspirin 325 mg delayed release tablet every 12 h as needed for pain. (one dose given the morning of 8.7.14)
17. Bisacodyl Suppository 10 mg rectal every four days as needed
18. Guiatuss liquid 1 tsp oral every 4–6 h as needed for cough
19. Maalox liquid 30 cc oral every 4–6 h as needed for indigestion
20. Meclizine HCl tablet 12.5 mg oral 2 tablets by mouth twice daily as needed for dizziness
21. Milk of Magnesia (Magnesium Hydroxide) suspension 400 mg/5 mL suspension 30 mL y mouth every third day as needed for constipation
22. Mucinex (Guaifenesin) tablet extended release 12 h 600 mg by mouth as need for congestion
23. Tramadol HCl tablet 50 mg by mouth every 8 h as needed for pain in thoracic spine

Side effects of medications

Mrs. Jones' physicians had the challenging task of prescribing multiple medications to treat her several coexisting medical problems, including her unstable and treatment-resistant anxiety and depression. In this difficult situation, Mrs. Jones' physicians elected to ease her severe anxiety symptoms with benzodiazepines: sedative-hypnotic medications that can effectively treat acute anxiety, but which are notorious for causing confusion. Benzodiazepines with a long half-life such as clorazepate are particularly likely to cause cognitive side effects, and can even cause a dementia-like syndrome.[38]

In Mrs. Jones' case, her severe anxiety had been inadequately controlled with the combination of citalopram (an antidepressant) and lorazepam (a benzodiazepine), so her doctor started clorazepate (another benzodiazepine, longer acting than lorazepam) while temporarily continuing the

[38] Olfson, M. et al. (2015). Benzodiazepine Use in the United States. JAMA Psychiatry 72(2):136–142.

lorazepam at a lower dose. Thus, on the day Mrs. Jones signed her new will, August 8, 2014, she received two concurrent benzodiazepines: clorazepate and lorazepam, alongside her numerous other scheduled medications.[39]

The table below highlights these and other medications deemed potentially inappropriate for elders according to the Beers criteria[40] that were prescribed to and taken by Mrs. Jones on August 8, 2014, the date of the will signing. Note that ataxia refers to a loss of control over bodily movements, syncope refers to fainting, and delirium refers to an acutely disturbed state of mind with restlessness and confusion of thought and speech.

Beers criteria: high risk medications

Medication taken by Mrs. Jones	Risks and possible effects[41]
Amiodarone	Toxicity, especially when combined with other medications
Citalopram	Ataxia, impaired psychomotor function, syncope, falls
Clorazepate	Ataxia, impaired psychomotor function, syncope, falls, adverse effects on the central nervous system, cognitive impairment, delirium, falls, fractures
Lorazepam	Ataxia, impaired psychomotor function, syncope, falls, adverse effects on the central nervous system, cognitive impairment, delirium, falls, fractures

Based on available evidence, the timeline on the next page shows some key psychotropic medication changes undergone by Mrs. Jones from July to September 2014. Of note, nursing staff documented that Clorazepate was temporarily unavailable from the pharmacy on, so Mrs. Jones did not receive her scheduled doses on Clorazepate on August 2, 3, and 4, 2014.[42]

39 Cumberland Care Center nursing home records (Bates stamped 1390—2143), 2013—4, p. 429—456.

40 American Geriatrics Society 2015 Beers Criteria Update Expert Panel (2015). American Geriatrics Society 2015 Updated Beers Criteria for Potentially Inappropriate Medication Use in Older Adults. J Am Geriatr Soc 63:2227—2246.

41 American Geriatrics Society 2015 Beers Criteria Update Expert Panel (2015). American Geriatrics Society 2015 Updated Beers Criteria for Potentially Inappropriate Medication Use in Older Adults. J Am Geriatr Soc 63:2227—2246.

42 Cumberland Care Center nursing home records (Bates stamped 1390—2143), 2013—4, p. 183, 433.

Mrs. Jones' medication changes, Jul–Sep 2014

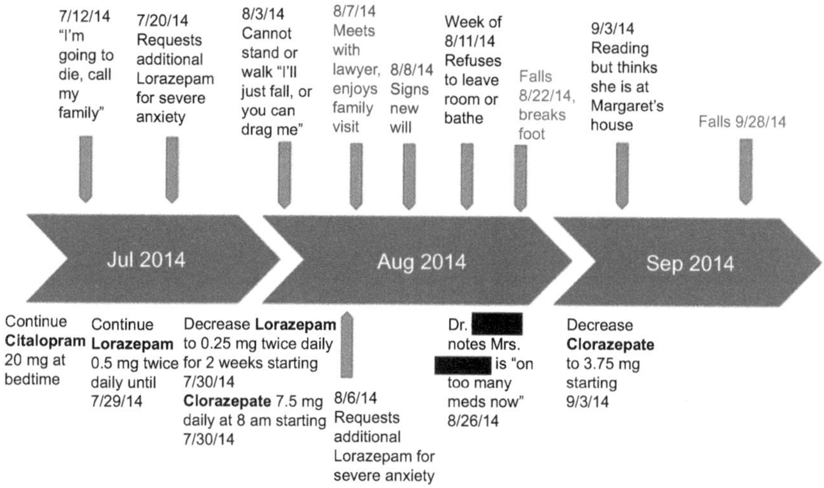

Further changes to medications

Within the next few weeks, Mrs. Jones underwent further changes to her psychotropic medication regimen, due to problematic side effects including multiple falls and concern about drug-drug interactions. Within a few weeks following August 8, 2014, Mrs. Jones' treating physicians eventually discontinued Lorazepam, halved the dose of Clorazepate, and replaced Citalopram with an alternative antidepressant having less potential for drug-drug interactions.[43]

Psychiatric and emotional issues

Mrs. Jones had a longstanding history of significant anxiety and depression, and continued to struggle with anxiety and depression until her death in April 2015. Her daughter Caitlyn Matthews testified that Mrs. Jones had been anxious all her life.[44]

Caitlyn Matthews also noted that Mrs. Jones had also suffered from hallucinations at the nursing home.[45] Indeed, records indicate that Mrs. Jones had brief episodes of psychotic symptoms (e.g. paranoia,

[43] Cumberland Care Center nursing home records (Bates stamped 1390–2143), 2013–4, p. 446–481.
[44] Deposition of Caitlyn Matthews/Roman (Co-Executor), 3/17/2017, 40–41.
[45] Deposition of Caitlyn Matthews/Roman (Co-Executor), 3/17/2017, p. 41.

hallucinations) while at the nursing home. However, based on the available records, it appears she did not suffer from chronic psychotic symptoms or a major psychotic disorder such as schizophrenia. Several of the nursing home records include a diagnosis of Psychosis/Confusion, but in my opinion Mrs. Jones' transient psychotic symptoms are best explained by a chronic progressive dementia process. Repeated defined episodes of delirium triggered by urinary tract infections or other medical or medication related issues could also have contributed to psychiatric symptoms. Dementia and delirium are much more likely than psychotic disorders in Mrs. Jones' case.

Psychiatric conditions

Mrs. Jones certainly struggled with chronic psychiatric conditions, particularly depression and anxiety for at least the last 20 years of her life.[46] In her final years, she also developed dementia (neurocognitive disorder).[47] Over many years, Mrs. Jones was treated with psychotropic medications including multiple antidepressants and benzodiazepines including lorazepam, alprazolam, and clorazepate. Records indicate that Mrs. Jones and her prescriber would periodically "wrestle with her Lorazepam" in the chronic course of her illness, indicating the difficulty of managing her chronic psychiatric symptoms.[48]

Mrs. Jones had a considerable experience of grief and loss, having been predeceased by her husband William Jones Sr., as well as by two of her sons, Richard Jones and William Jones Jr. These difficult losses likely played a role in Mrs. Jones' depression and anxiety complaints. Experiences of grief and loss likely made Mrs. Jones more worried about preserving her relationship with her son Alexander Jones and daughter Caitlyn Matthews, and made her more dependent on them and others.

Mrs. Jones' institutionalization likely induced and exaggerated dependent tendencies and brought about regressed personality characteristics. A dependent stance can make a person more passive, and more likely to go along with someone else's ideas. This is significant considering Mrs. Jones' special relationship with her son Alexander Jones.[49]

[46] Cumberland Hospital medical records (Bates stamped 123—747), 2011—4, p. 272; Deposition of Caitlyn Matthews/Roman (Co-Executor), 3/17/2017, p. 40—41; Cumberland Care Center nursing home records (Bates stamped 1390—2143), 2013—4, p. 187.

[47] Cumberland Care Center nursing home records (Bates stamped 1390—2143), 2013—4, p. 22.

[48] Cumberland Care Center nursing home records (Bates stamped 1390—2143), 2013—4, p. 47.

[49] Deposition of Marlene Jones (Mother of Plaintiffs and daughter-in-law of Decedent, Carolyn Jones), 3/17/2017, p. 38—40, 48.

Criteria for testamentary capacity

Evidence from available records throws light on Mrs. Jones' impaired mental ability at the time the 2014 will was made. Mrs. Jones suffered from dementia, emotional vulnerabilities, physical weakness and infirmity. The criteria below are used to determine testamentary capacity, the ability to make a valid will:

Knows a will is being made

The available records do not clearly indicate that Mrs. Jones knew and understood that a new will was being made. Cumberland Care Center staff documented on August 6, 2014 that Mrs. Jones said she planned to wake up early the next morning because the lawyer was coming to her room, which suggests that Mrs. Jones had a basic understanding of the situation. However, no further documentation is available regarding Mrs. Jones' specific knowledge of the events on the days the will was made and signed.

Knows the kind and extent of her property

Mrs. Jones had an undivided one-half interest in the family real estate.[50] However, her lawyer's notes from August 7, 2014, the day of Mrs. Jones' meeting with the lawyer, Alexander Jones and Caitlyn Matthews indicate that Mrs. Jones would be dividing an estate of 400 acres in half, leaving 200 acres each to Alexander Jones and Caitlyn Matthews.[51] In fact, the inheritance plan in the will Mrs. Jones signed the next day was much more complicated, since the land was already partially accounted for, and could not simply be split in half as the lawyer appears to have discussed with Mrs. Jones based on the handwritten notes. The complicated nature of this situation, along with Mrs. Jones' progressing dementia and frailty, makes it more likely than not that Mrs. Jones did not recognize the kind and extent of her property. Mrs. Jones could not understand what she was signing when she signed the 2014 will.

[50] Answers to Interrogatories which were executed and served by plaintiffs, 12/7/2016, p. 14.
[51] Exhibit 40, see Deposition Exhibits 20–42, 3/17/2017.

Can identify and remember those persons she would naturally give her property to

Mrs. Jones suffered from dementia at the time she signed the 2014 will. Difficulties recalling family history and the identity of family members would have a direct impact on Mrs. Jones' ability to recall those persons she would naturally give her property to, presumably her children and grandchildren. From the time William Jones Senior passed away, Mrs. Jones repeatedly said that the estate plan put in place prior to William's death would never be changed.[52]

Knows how she wants to distribute her property

Mrs. Jones thought she had the right to give away 400 acres, but in fact the 2014 will outlines a more complicated situation.[53] I am aware of no available evidence that shows Mrs. Jones understood the particular disposition plan outlined in her 2014 will. In my opinion, given her advancing dementia, Mrs. Jones would not have been able to read and understand a detailed plan of this nature.

Criteria for undue influence

Undue influence involves the substitution of one person's wishes for another's. At the time Mrs. Jones' 2014 will was made, she was clearly susceptible to undue influence. Below, I will list several indicators of undue influence and provide information about the presence of each of these indicators in this case.

Dominance over the testator

Mrs. Jones had a special relationship with her son Alexander Jones. She was completely dependent on him, his wife Stacy Jones, and Mrs. Jones' daughter Caitlyn Matthews to manage financial affairs.

Family members testified that Alexander Jones would at times show intimidating behavior toward his mother Mrs. Jones, would bully her, had a hot temper, would scream and holler.[54] Family members also testified that

52 Answers to Interrogatories which were executed and served by plaintiffs, 12/7/2016, p. 14.
53 Exhibit 3, see Deposition Exhibits 1–19, 3/17/2017.
54 Deposition of Timothy Jones (Plaintiff), 3/17/2017, p. 48.

Alexander Jones would use intimidation directed Mrs. Jones about her finances, told her to sell land, had a temper, would become upset and bang his fists.[55]

Whether the condition of the testator's mind was subject to such dominance

Available records indicate that Mrs. Jones was frail and vulnerable, physically, mentally and emotionally, suffering from dementia, and taking multiple medications. Throughout her lifetime, and at the time the 2014 will was signed, Mrs. Jones struggled with anxiety and depression. Records suggest Mrs. Jones may have felt intimidated by her son Alexander Jones, yet during the two 2014 will related meetings at the nursing home on August 7 and 8, 2014, the will co-executors Alexander Jones and Caitlyn Matthews remained in the room. Mrs. Jones did not speak with the lawyer alone.[56]

Whether the distribution of the testator's property is unnatural, unjust or unreasonable

Available records indicate that for 15 years, it was Mrs. Jones' intention to distribute her estate according to the terms outlined in her 1999 will, executed during the lifetime of her husband William Jones Sr.[57] The 2014 will was inconsistent with Mrs. Jones' established prior wishes regarding the disposition of her estate.[58] It is the province of the court to decide whether the co-executors benefited unduly from the new will.

The activity of the person charged with exercising the undue influence and whether the person had the opportunity and frame of mind to exercise undue influence

Evidence in this case indicates that Alexander Jones, a co-executor and beneficiary of the 2014 will, was active in obtaining the services of the attorney who drew up the 2014 will. Alexander Jones also arranged for the two meetings at the nursing home during which the new will was discussed and signed, then Alexander Jones picked up the revised will document from the attorney's office and brought it to his mother Mrs. Jones in the nursing

55 Deposition of Brian Jones (Plaintiff), 3/17/2017, p. 30.

56 Deposition of Caitlyn Matthews/Roman (Co-Executor), 3/17/2017, p. 39.

57 Answers to Interrogatories which were executed and served by plaintiffs, 12/7/2016, p. 14.

58 Deposition of Marlene Jones (Mother of Plaintiffs and daughter-in-law of Decedent, Carolyn Jones), 3/17/2017, p. 36.

home so she could sign it. Alexander Jones then brought the signed will back to the attorney's office.

The intelligence or lack of intelligence of the testator

At the time of the signing of the 2014 will, Mrs. Jones suffered from dementia which was moderate to severe in degree. Available records do not contain specific information about her intelligence prior to onset of dementia.

Whether the testator was physically or mentally weak

Mrs. Jones was extremely frail, physically weak and feeble, suffering from multiple medical problems and taking numerous prescribed medications. Mrs. Jones was mentally weak. She suffered from dementia, depression and anxiety. She was completely dependent on her children Alexander Jones and Caitlyn Matthews for management of her finances and property. She was completely dependent on nursing home staff for activities of daily living, medical care, meal preparation and other basic activities of daily living.

Whether the person charged with exercising undue influence was the controlling party in a confidential relationship with the testator (gained complete confidence of testator, purports to act or advise with only the interest of testator in mind)

Mrs. Jones was completely financially dependent on her son Alexander Jones and trusted him with all her financial matters. This dependency clearly created an opportunity for Alexander Jones to control the testamentary act. Though Mrs. Jones trusted Alexander Jones to act and advise with only the interest of Mrs. Jones in mind, family members remarked that in fact, Mrs. Jones would kowtow to Alexander Jones, and that Alexander Jones financially took advantage of Mrs. Jones regarding the farm rental. Checks were written for Alexander Jones' benefit from Mrs. Jones' bank account.[59] Mrs. Jones also trusted her daughter Caitlyn Matthews to help with finances, however Caitlyn Matthews testified that her own understanding of family financial matters was minimal.[60]

59 Answers to Interrogatories which were executed and served by plaintiffs, 12/7/2016, p. 15; Deposition of Alexander Jones (Co-Executor), 3/17/2017, p. 58.

60 Deposition of Caitlyn Matthews/Roman (Co-Executor), 3/17/2017, p. 12–14.

Other facts or circumstances shown by the evidence which may have any bearing on the question

Mrs. Jones, at the age of 95 when she signed the 2014 will, was in an extremely weak state, medically ill, suffering from dementia, emotionally fragile and completely dependent on others for even the most basic activities of daily living. She was clearly susceptible to undue influence.

Opinions

Mrs. Jones did not have the mental ability to make a will in August 2014

Based on the available evidence, it is my opinion to a reasonable degree of medical certainty that Mrs. Jones lacked testamentary capacity at the time of the signing of her 2014 will. In my opinion, the available evidence indicates that Mrs. Jones did not understand what she was signing when she signed her 2014 will. The available records demonstrate she was in an extremely weak condition, physically, mentally and emotionally.

As discussed above, the following factors interfered with her mental ability to make a will:

1. Dementia
2. Medical illness and physical frailty
3. Polypharmacy (multiple medications)
4. Emotional vulnerability

Aside from the quarterly BIMS assessments which indicated moderate to severe cognitive impairment, I am aware of no other evidence of a formal assessment of her mental capacities, such as a standardized mental status evaluation or a neuropsychological evaluation. In addition, it is unclear whether Mrs. Jones had appropriate accommodations for her severe hearing and vision problems (glasses and hearing aids) during the meetings that took place.

Mrs. Jones was susceptible to undue influence at the time her 2014 will was made

Based on the available evidence, it is my opinion to a reasonable degree of medical certainty that Mrs. Jones was susceptible to undue influence by the co-executors of the 2014 will, Alexander Jones and Caitlyn Matthews. Mrs.

Jones' mental and physical weakness indicates that the intentions and purpose of the 2014 will were not Mrs. Jones'.

A review of the available data in this case makes it clear that Mrs. Jones was susceptible to undue influence prior to her death. She was mentally and physically weak, suffering from serious medical problems and frailty. Mrs. Jones suffered from significant cognitive impairment and was diagnosed with dementia. Medical personnel were noticing cognitive impairment consistent with dementia for at least a year prior to the signing of the 2014 will, and Mrs. Jones' progressive dementia and extremely low level of functioning was documented in the months preceding and following the will. Mrs. Jones' emotional and cognitive problems put her in a vulnerable state. Her dependence on her son Alexander Jones and daughter Caitlyn Matthews provided the opportunity for the subversion of her free will in the disposition of her estate according to the terms of the 2014 will.

Sample report: competency to stand trial (CST)*

The report example may not contain all the elements that can be included in a criminal forensic neuropsychological report, or be written in the preferred style of the reader's jurisdiction. The reader should consult with the courts and more experienced forensic colleagues to ensure that the report they write meets local statutory and regulatory requirements as well as conforming to the preferred report styles for the particular setting and particular legal question.

Hon._______, Judge ____________

Judicial District Court.

RE: report concerning Ms. Doe defendant, competency to stand trial case no. ([state] v. A. B.)

Dear Judge_________:

You have asked that I evaluate Ms. Doe and report to you regarding.

(1) her competence to stand trial and
(2) if not currently competent, whether or not there is a substantial probability that, with or without treatment, she will attain competence within the foreseeable future.

I am able to supply the comments and opinions below, based upon records and information received, personal examination, and my training, background, and experience. The methods used and materials reviewed are those routinely relied upon by forensic psychiatrists in matters such as these.

Materials reviewed

Materials supplied by your office: (list) (date) Psychological testing done at my request by Dr. _________ Interviews and examinations (list).

My background, training, and experience in medicine, psychiatry, and forensic psychiatry Qualifications I am a clinical and forensic psychiatrist

* Adapted from Dr. Reid (Developing a forensic practice), Donders (Neuropsychological Report Writing).

with training and experience in medicine, psychiatry, and forensic psychiatry. My qualifications are further outlined in the curriculum vitae which has been supplied to your office.

Notification/informed consent

Ms. Doe was informed that my psychological and neuropsychological evaluation had been ordered by the court and that I was being retained by the prosecuting attorney's office. She was informed that nothing we discussed would remain confidential, and that information she provided during our clinical interview and the test results from my examination of her would become a part of my report, to be used in upcoming proceedings. She was informed that a copy of any report I produced would be sent to her attorneys, the prosecuting attorneys, and the court. Ms. De indicated that she understood the purpose of the evaluation, and the limitations of confidentiality of our interview and the testing I conducted.

Background

Ms. Doe is a woman with an extensive history of psychiatric hospitalizations for acute manic episodes of bipolar disorder. Historically, she presented as acutely psychotic and out of contact with reality with grandiose, paranoid delusions, expansive mood, pressured speech, flight of ideas (rapid flow of the mind from one thought to another) and irritability, hostility, and combativeness. These are all classic symptoms of the manic state of bipolar disorder. In previous competency evaluations that I reviewed, some of these symptoms remained, particularly delusional, disorganized thinking and impaired judgment, necessitating the doctors to conclude that she was not competent to proceed to trial.

Findings

At the present time, Ms. Doe's clinical condition shows considerable improvement. She was rational, logical, cooperative, in good spirits, and recognized her previous delusional and grandiose symptoms. It could not be reliably determined if her statements regarding her educational attainment and book authorship are truthful or not. If not, she may still manifest some degree of grandiose delusional thinking or she could simply be lying. But, as will be discussed below, nonetheless I believe her to be competent to proceed to trial.

My current diagnosis is bipolar disorder, type I, in remission.

Ms. Doe is aware of her current surroundings, the hospital building, city, state, and her doctors. She was aware of the date and time. She knows the president and vice president. She remembered me from a previous examination of several months ago.

Ms. Doe correctly stated the charges against her. She correctly stated the judge, the roles of the judge, prosecutor defense attorney, and jury. She understands the term "plea bargain" and the consequences. She understands she has the right to testify or not.

Opinions

The following opinions are offered to a reasonable degree of medical and psychiatric certainty, as I understand the meaning of that phrase. Please note that my opinions are not intended to usurp the authority of the trier of fact in actually determining competency.

These understandings were also apparent in the most recent previous examination for competency conducted in April of 2018. But at that time, she was felt to be too disorganized, delusional and unrealistic to adequately participate in her own defense.

At the time, however, Ms. Doe is far less disturbed, shows considerably less delusional thinking, and is rational, coherent and logical. Ms. Doe demonstrates sufficient factual and rational understanding of courtroom procedures and of her legal case for competency to proceed to trial. She can assist her attorney to a reasonable degree in her own defense, and her mental disorder will not impede her from doing so.

Ms. Doe's psychiatric condition and level of competency appear stable as of the date of my evaluation. It should be noted that she is being treated by Dr. _____ (a psychiatrist) and is taking psychiatric medication which improves her thinking and her contact with reality.

If (a) she continues such treatment and medication, I have no reason to believe that her level of competence will deteriorate substantially between the time of my evaluation and the time of trial, assuming no extraordinary delay.

If (b) she stops taking those medications, her level of competence could deteriorate within days or weeks, and she may or may not become incompetent to stand trial.

Clinician's guide to the geriatric forensic interview*

Here is an outline of some of the key information clinicians may consider for a geriatric forensic interview. This template is not prescriptive. It is provided to act as a starting point and guide for clinicians.

Pre-assessment preparation

- Who is involved in this case?
- Do I have a conflict of interest or a bias issue?
- Is the court or litigants involved?
- What is the legal question? Why is this question being raised?
- What is the time frame of interest?
- Am I appropriately qualified to assess this?
- Is an evaluation/report requested?
- When does the evaluation/report need to be completed?

Legal question

- What is the legal standard in question?
- Are there functional elements to consider?

For retrospective evaluation

- What is the history of the case?
- What time frame is being considered?
- Are records adequate to address the question being asked?

The geriatric forensic interview

Informed consent

- Why is the evaluation requested? Procedures involved in evaluation? Potential risks?

* Adapted from: Capacity Worksheet for Psychologists, in Assessment of Older Adults with Diminished Capacity: A Handbook for Psychologists by the ABA Commission on Law and Aging and the American Psychological Association (2008).

- Potential benefits? Uses of the report?
- Limits on privacy and confidentiality?

Records review

- Medical records
- Diagnoses
- Laboratory Tests
- Imaging
- Other Treatments
- Medications
- Legal records
- Documents filed in the court
- Financial statements
- HCP/POAHC documents
- Other Records

Collateral interviews

- Family
- Staff/Professional Caregivers
- Other

Accommodating and enhancing capacity during the assessment

- Assess recent events and losses, such as bereavement
- Explore medical factors such as nutrition, medications, hydration
- Select tests inconsideration of cultural and language issues
- Administer tests in primary language
- Select tests that are validated for the age of the person
- Assess ability to read and accommodate reading difficulties
- Adjust seating, lighting
- Use visual and hearing aids
- Consider fatigue; Take breaks; Use multiple testing sessions

Cognitive evaluation

- Sensory intactness
- Motor function
- Processing speed
- Attention and concentration

- Memory
- Language comprehension
- Communication
- Calculation
- Verbal Reasoning
- Visual-Spatial ability
- Executive Function

Psychiatric/emotional factors

- Disorganized Thinking
- Hallucinations
- Delusions
- Anxiety
- Mania
- Depressed Mood
- Insight
- Impulsivity
- Noncompliance

Values

- Preferences for how decisions made?
- And by whom?
- Preferences for living setting?
- Goals including self-assessment of quality of life?
- Concerns, fears, preferences, religious views?
- Preferences for spending and saving?
- Impact of culture, age, sexual orientation, diversity?
- Views about guardianship (if applicable)?

Risks

- Is the risk new or old?
- How serious is the risk?
- How imminent is the risk?
- What is the risk of harm to self?
- To others?
- Are there concrete instances of failure?
- How objective is the assessment of risk?

Findings/opinions

- Opinions
- Diagnoses and Prognoses
  - What diagnoses account for the deficits?
  - Can conditions be treated?
  - Are deficits likely to get better, worse or stay the same?
  - When should the older adult be re-evaluated?

For capacity/guardianship

Capacity framework

- The functional abilities constituent to the capacity
- Cognitive abilities, psychiatric/emotional functioning, and medical diagnoses and prognosis, as they relate to the functional abilities;
- Specific risks of the capacity situation.
- Has capacity for decision/task in question Lacks capacity for decision/task in question
- Has marginal capacity for decision/task in question (if the case is not being adjudicated, recommended course of action)

Steps to enhance capacity

Would the Older Adult benefit from:

- Education, training, or rehabilitation?
- Mental health treatment?
- Occupational, physical, or other therapy?
- Home and/or social services?
- Assistive devices or accommodations?
- Medical treatment, operation or procedure?
- Other?

Montreal cognitive assessment (MoCA)

The MoCA is a cognitive screening tool that allows quick assessment of a patient's cognitive health across multiple domains. Multiple versions of the MoCA are available.

Clinicians must follow instructions when administering the MoCA, to ensure standardization of the testing procedures. A Training and Certification program for the MoCA will become mandatory as of September 1, 2019. See www.mocatest.org for details.

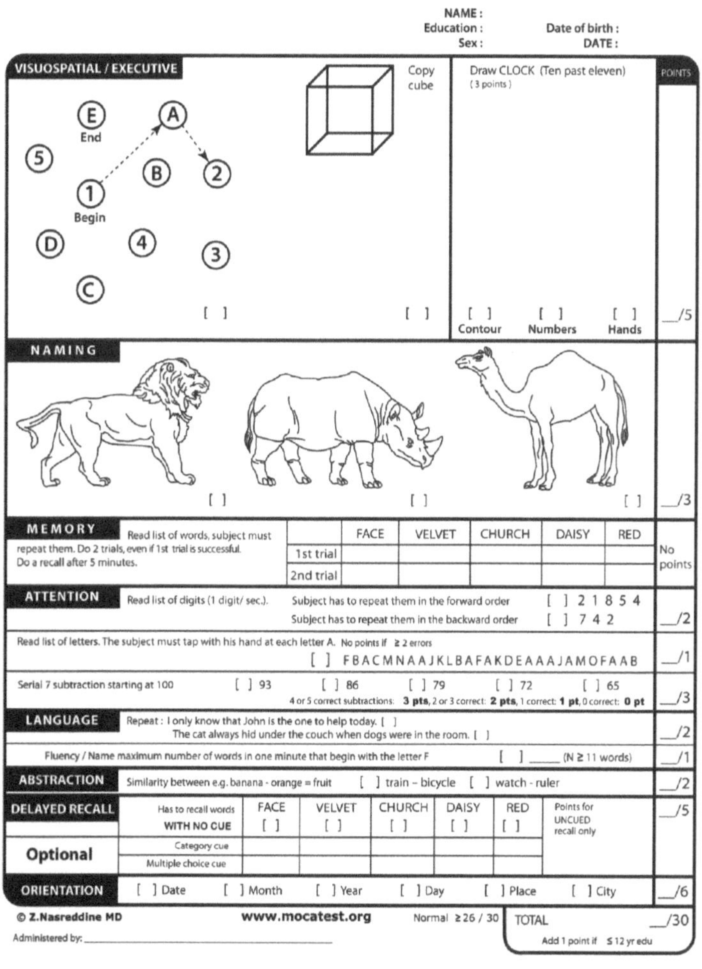

NAME :
Education : Date of birth :
Sex : DATE :

POINTS

VISUOSPATIAL / EXECUTIVE

[ ]

Copy cube [ ]

Draw CLOCK (Ten past eleven) (3 points)

[ ] Contour [ ] Numbers [ ] Hands

___/5

NAMING

[ ] [ ] [ ]

___/3

MEMORY Read list of words, subject must repeat them. Do 2 trials, even if 1st trial is successful. Do a recall after 5 minutes.

	FACE	VELVET	CHURCH	DAISY	RED
1st trial					
2nd trial					

No points

ATTENTION Read list of digits (1 digit/ sec.).
Subject has to repeat them in the forward order [ ] 2 1 8 5 4
Subject has to repeat them in the backward order [ ] 7 4 2
___/2

Read list of letters. The subject must tap with his hand at each letter A. No points if ≥ 2 errors
[ ] F B A C M N A A J K L B A F A K D E A A A J A M O F A A B
___/1

Serial 7 subtraction starting at 100 [ ] 93 [ ] 86 [ ] 79 [ ] 72 [ ] 65
4 or 5 correct subtractions: **3 pts**, 2 or 3 correct: **2 pts**, 1 correct: **1 pt**, 0 correct: **0 pt**
___/3

LANGUAGE Repeat : I only know that John is the one to help today. [ ]
The cat always hid under the couch when dogs were in the room. [ ]
___/2

Fluency / Name maximum number of words in one minute that begin with the letter F [ ] _____ (N ≥ 11 words)
___/1

ABSTRACTION Similarity between e.g. banana - orange = fruit [ ] train – bicycle [ ] watch - ruler
___/2

DELAYED RECALL		FACE	VELVET	CHURCH	DAISY	RED	
	Has to recall words **WITH NO CUE**	[ ]	[ ]	[ ]	[ ]	[ ]	Points for UNCUED recall only
Optional	Category cue						
	Multiple choice cue						

___/5

ORIENTATION [ ] Date [ ] Month [ ] Year [ ] Day [ ] Place [ ] City
___/6

© Z.Nasreddine MD   **www.mocatest.org**   Normal ≥26 / 30   TOTAL ___/30
Add 1 point if ≤ 12 yr edu

Administered by: ________________

Copyright Z. Nasreddine MD. Reproduced with permission

Index

'*Note:* Page numbers followed by "f" indicate figures, "t" indicate tables and "b" indicate boxes.'

B

C

Kolibri 360 GmbH
Ferdinand-Jühlke-Straße 7
99095 Erfurt, Deutschland
produktsicherheit@kolibri360.de